For Health's Sake

A Cancer Survivor's Cookbook

Other Books by MyLinda Butterworth:

JUST 24 DAYS TILL CHRISTMAS, Act 1: Old and New Frogazoom!

For Health's Sake

A Cancer Survivor's Cookbook

MyLinda Butterworth

Day to Day Enterprises 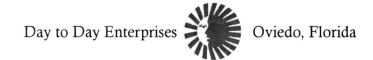 Oviedo, Florida

Library of Congress Catalog Card Number: 99-66238
ISBN: 1-890905-04-6 softcover
ISBN: 1-890905-18-6 hardcover

Printed in the United States of America
10 9 8 7 6 5 4 3 2 1

PUBLISHER'S NOTE
The ideas, procedures and suggestions contained in this book are
not intended as a substitute for consulting with your physician. We
recommend that all matters regarding your health should be deferred
to a medical doctor who has a good working knowledge and practice
of nutrition.

Published by
Day to Day Enterprises
1721 Canoe Creek Rd., Oviedo, Florida 32766-8533
books@daytodayenterprises.com
http://www.daytodayenterprises.com

This book is dedicated to my husband,
Michael R Butterworth,
who stood by me through it all and supported and
encouraged my decisions. My life would truly be
nothing without him and his endless love for me.

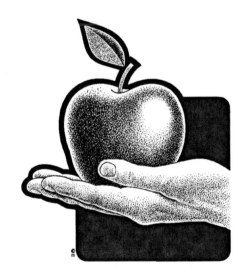

Special Thanks

I want to thank God, for his love, guidance and healing touch in my life. To my parents, Bob and Linda Day, who never let me give up and listened to my unending whining about life's little battles. To the following friends; Linda Humphrey who is willing to read and edit my books; Paula Kalinoski who loaned me her home for the taste testing party and for her unending encouragement to write; Lisa Potter who is always there for me; JoAnne Abercrombie who was willing to help me revise some of the recipes so that they were more vegan/vegetarian and loaned me numerous books and tapes in my quest for enlightenment on nutrition; Evie Knecht and her family who were willing to be my guinea pigs on numerous tasting adventures; and all the people who were willing to make and taste recipes for the taste testing party. Without all of you this project would have been dead in the water.

Contents

Preface ix
Forward xi
Introduction xiii
Chapter 1: Cancer; A Learning Process 1
Chapter 2: Healing: Body and Soul 11
Chapter 3: Grains of Knowledge 23
Chapter 4: Fresh and Fruity 25
Chapter 5: Veggie Power 29
Chapter 6: Bowled Over by Beans 33
Chapter 7: Seasonings by Herb 35
Chapter 8: Mooove Over Dairy 39
Chapter 9: Get off the Fat-Go-Round 43
Chapter 10: The Truth About Sweeteners 47
Chapter 11: Oh No, I'm Out of ... A Guide to Substitutions 49
Appetizers, Beverages and So Forth 54
    Soul Snacks 55
    Appetizers 55
    Beverages 60
    So Forth 66
Soups and Salads 75
    Soul Snacks 76
    Soups 77
    Salads 84
Breads 95
    Soul Snacks 96
Fruits and Veggies 115
    Soul Snacks 116
    Fruits 117
    Veggies 119
Main Dishes 131
    Soul Snacks 132
Sauces and Dressings 153
    Soul Snacks 154
    Sauces 155
    Salad Dressings 158
Sweet Treats 163
    Soul Snacks 164
    Cookies 165
    Cakes, Frostings and Fillings 178
    Pies and Pastry 189
    Desserts 194
    Candy 197
My Favorite Books 202
Bibliography 203
Index 205
About the Author 213

Preface

When I first wrote *For Health's Sake* in 1981, the world looked at nutrition and diet through rose colored glasses. That is to say there really wasn't much out there to help you become healthy; body and soul. The health revolution was just beginning and what books were out there were sometimes very radical or just plain timid. I began my venture into nutritious eating almost blindfolded, with just a little bit of information to guide me. Since then there has been an explosion of research and know-how released to the general public.

I would call myself a student of nutrition. Not someone who takes classes at the university in the chemistry of food, but one who is always looking, reading and siphoning all the information I can about what's new in the world of nutrition and cancer. I keep files on the subject. I don't think you can ever stop learning. Because of that and the encouragement of many friends I have revised my original book. Given it a face lift and a lot of thought and information about the foods you eat. Then it is up to you to decide if what I have to offer is of value to you or just a bunch of beans that make you toot.

The recipes in this book have been created with taste in mind first and low-calorie, low-fat and low-sugar coming in second. Many of these recipes have been used in my home since I first started to make dietary changes in 1979 and have changed little since then. This book has been revised because in the eighteen years since I originally wrote this book, nutritional information has changed. Back in 1981 when the first book was written, sugar was the enemy and fat was just an annoyance. Life has changed since then and this book now reflects the healthy changes that have emerged.

At the end of each recipe, you will find important nutrition information, the calorie count of each serving; the amount in grams, of fat, satfat (saturated fat), protein, carbohydrates, cholesterol and sodium. The nutritional analysis is based on the computer program MasterCook produced by Sierra, with input of product nutrient information from various brand-name companies mention in the book. These analysis are correct to the best of our knowledge, but should only be used as a guide. Please note that whenever a choice has been given, the ingredient listed first is the one used in the calculation. If you choose to use the other ingredient listed that the analysis will change.

My only prayer for those who read these pages is that they will give the changes they make in their food consumption a chance to work. Nothing worthwhile ever happened overnight. Your tastebuds will change and you will start tasting the foods you eat, because they have less fat, sugar and salt. One day you will be offered a fancy cookie or dessert you really want and you will take a bite and say, "Man this is too sweet," and at that point you will have arrived at success. Knowing that what changes you have made, do make a difference. It will work and you will feel stronger and happier because you feel good inside and out. I'm living proof!

I wrote this book to be used FOR HEALTH'S SAKE and yours. Enjoy!

Foreword

MyLinda was seen in our medical office in July of 1979, having returned from a two-month trip in Europe with her husband, healthy, vibrant, alive, and was seeing one of my partners simply to evaluate some irregular bleeding. At that time a mass was felt by my associate in her left side. Pregnancy test was obtained to rule out a possible tubal pregnancy. The pregnancy tests were all negative. Because of the size of the mass and the patient's age, we felt that she most likely had a benign tumor and so were not overly concerned. At that time, we decided to proceed with a diagnostic laparoscopy, which is a way to minimally invasively examine the pelvis.

Twenty years later, I can still recall quite well the procedure because of my surprise that a 22-year-old with a pelvis that was full of carcinoma. Her left ovary was markedly enlarged with numerous cancerous growths, which had attached to her large bowel. She had a growth in the area known as the cu-de-sac behind the uterus. The right ovary was also involved. At the time, we did washings of fluid in her pelvis for malignant cells, which were also positive. A report was sent to the pathologist who gave us the bad news during the laparoscopy that this indeed was malignant. A decision was made to proceed with a total abdominal hysterectomy, removal of both ovaries, thus eliminating any chance that MyLinda could have children of her own.

I can still recall my thoughts at the time about what was important and what wasn't. Here was a young person who had just returned from a great vacation in Europe with the world on a string. She goes to sleep for what we thought would be a simple procedure. She awakes to find out that she has a life threatening condition. I remember thinking that things that were so important, you master card bill and all the little quirks in life that bother us day in and day out were no longer important. I can also recall thinking that if they weren't important after we found out she had cancer, why were they important before she had cancer. I think about this often.

Cancer of the ovary is staged in four stages, I-IV. Her stage was III-C. I placed two silastic catheters in her peritoneal cavity and being recently out of residency, I elected to use radioactive phosphorous in an effort to battle the cancer. She tolerated this well. She recovered quite well from the surgery as would be expected in a young person. MyLinda was referred for further consultation with an oncologist, but after one treatment, elected not to continue chemotherapy.

MyLinda's victory over cancer of the ovary has certainly been an inspiration to me and to others. When I counsel a patient that I see currently who has ovarian cancer, her success always comes to mind and gives me hope for patients. MyLinda has been and continues to be proactive in her approach to disease. She has used diet, a very positive mental approach, and a supportive family, that has all contributed to her success.

I hope her book will serve as an inspiration for people who are facing the same demon that she has conquered.

With warmest personal regards,

Phil

David P. Roe, M.D.
State of Franklin Healthcare Associates, PLLC
Medical Center Obstetrics and Gynecology, P.C.
Johnson City, Tennessee

Introduction

I am pleased to write about simple foods and good choices that give us sustaining energy, health and wholeness. The food we eat each day is where we get our daily ration of energy. Our choices can give us the stamina to not only endure but make the most of what each day brings. Simple foods cooked simply are the key to our health, happiness and peace. What we eat becomes our blood. The quality of our blood directly determines the quality of our health.

MyLinda has a personal triumph to share — a story to tell, as do so many of us. My children had chronic ear infections. It always started as croup that moved in bronchitis and then to ear infections. Frequent visits to their doctor for antibiotics never addressed the real issues. I became a single parent who struggled with health problems-my children's and my own. When I got sick there was no financial support to allow me time to rest and recuperate. I went to work with pneumonia for three weeks. A co-worker gave me the phone number of a man named Jorge Marquez who used whole foods and herbs for healing. I followed his instructions and was well in three days, ready to return to work. I was asked to stop all dairy and meat products. I gave myself ginger compresses and ate miso soup daily. I was so impressed with my recovery that I decided to put my girls on the same diet. In almost 20 years since that decision, we have not had a single ear infection or case of croup, bronchitis or pneumonia.

As the weeks and months passed from my initial healing, I began to notice my monthly cycles became easier. This was such a relief compared to the difficulty I had endured during my old way of eating. This opened my eyes to a whole new world of information and experience. As with anything we discover, I began to share what little I knew with favorable results and raves of joy from people, who suddenly found new energy, lost weight and felt happier. They requested classes and I began studying, taking and giving vegan vegetarian cooking classes. I have learned how powerful it is. My gratitude for this knowledge and my passion to share what I know is great.

I know have many friends who chose food and exercise as their way of healing and they are here many long and happy years after they were told they would not be. They are vibrant, energetic, happy people who share with others their knowledge and their stories. When we find a good thing we share it. The proof is in the pudding!

This is what MyLinda has done in her cookbook of choices, sharing with us many good recipes. I want to thank MyLinda for all the hard work and the many long hours she has devoted to researching and bringing this book together for all of us. She has always had great energy and a creative gift that she is always happy to share in extending her knowledge to others. All who know her have felt blessed to learn as a result of her great and endless talents. When you experience the despair of a serious degenerative disease and recover through this miraculous healing process, your example becomes powerful and gives hope to those who stand in need. Power that gives us the ability to make choices without fear or guilt or lack of knowledge — all of which can harm us. Ignorance can have a very high price.

MyLinda has given us lots of useful and practical information with a multitutde of good choices, healthy choices. For some of the possibility of existing on a whole foods diet depends on being convinced we could find good meals that taste good and don't harm us. The evidence is in and it is clear, if we make good choices we can restore and preserve our health. The entrance to transformation is sometimes through the rice field and sometimes through the gingerbread house. As cooks we create it all. Especially fun are desserts! They make us all the same age. If we study, make joy our aim and love our craft we can make edible monuments to delight our families and ourselves. Just watch your stock go up at home.

As you practice, your personal power and expression will flourish. You will then make good choices that will create good meals that will produce a wonderful energy. This positive energy is then passed along to our children who pass it to their children and life goes on abundantly as God intended, long, healthy and happy. When we avail ourselves of these wonderful blessings we can do the work we are here to do so much more effectively and with greater satisfaction. Start a garden, educate yourselves and make wise choices.

We are worth every good choice we make.

JoAnne Abercombie
Chef and Instructor
The Greater Life
July 31, 1999

Chapter One

Cancer: A Learning Process

When you're twenty-two years old you think your life is just beginning and the world is your oyster, or at least that is what you're led to believe. I was no different. I mean I was a newlywed of one year and I was completely in love with Mike, my husband. We had just returned from an incredible six weeks jaunt in Europe for our first wedding anniversary. I was one semester away from graduating from college. I was young, energetic, enthusiastic about life and in good health (or at least I thought so), who could ask for more? Could you?

With so much going for me, it seemed like a perfect time to begin a family, so I did what most would do, I went to my gynecologist to make sure all my parts were working properly. The group of doctors I visited was Scholls, Cone, Roe and Dunkleberger in Johnson City, Tennessee where we were currently living. They were a nice bunch of doctors and I had always felt at ease visiting with them (at least as much as one can). So why should my visit this time be any different? I had just been there 8 weeks ago and Dr. Scholls had given me some birth control pills to try and straighten out my menstrual periods so I could start planning to get pregnant. I always wanted a big family and why shouldn't I? I was the oldest of eight and Mike the oldest of four. Mike and I wanted five children; we had even picked out their names, Ammon, Brant, Chantel, Evette and Devin. Anyway as it is with all these type doctor visits, it entailed a pelvic exam (I really hate them), it was no different, or so I thought.

Dr. Scholls was my physician that day (he always reminded me of a kindly old grandfather); he was from the old school, so that meant when he did my pelvic exam he always had his eyes closed. Today, he did not have any smiles for me and I winced in pain a few times when he did some of his prodding. He wasn't quite sure what he was feeling and I didn't quite like how it felt. Since the uterus was slightly swollen there was a chance of pregnancy, but it was only slight, also there was an ovary that he felt might have a cyst on it. He wanted another opinion so he had me set another appointment to come in and see Dr. Roe.

The next day I came back to the office and this time I would see Dr. Roe. He told me that my Pap smear had come back negative and that he was pleased about that. Then he proceeded to give me the same exam I had yesterday. Dr. Roe tries to be pleasant and talk to me while he is giving me this unpleasant exam. When he is finished, he snaps off his little rubber gloves and says; "Now don't you move, I want to get Dr. Dunkleberger in here to see what he thinks. I will be back in a minute." Now when your doctors give you the 'I'm not sure look,' and leaves to get someone else for a third opinion, your mind starts racing.

With the completion of the third pelvic exam I am just a little stressed and sore. Dr. Roe tells me to get dressed and then leaves the room. I slowly climbed off the exam table and got dressed. I don't understand what is going on. I felt fine. What could possibly be wrong with me? I began to think about my life. I never smoked, used drugs or drank alcohol, I had been physically active all my life and had just finished working the past nine months as a manager of a figure salon so I was in pretty good shape. I ate a good diet (even though I did enjoy a good bar of candy or bowl of ice cream from time to time), all in all I couldn't think of anything that should cause me any concern.

A knock came on the door and I said, "Come on in." The nurse asked me to follow her down to Dr. Scholls office. I bolstered myself up and walked confidently down the hall to his office and sat down in the large overstuffed leather chair across from his desk. A few minutes later Dr. Scholls strolled into the room and sat down, and started to glance through my charts. He then raised his head, looked me straight in the eyes and said, "MyLinda, I don't think we have anything to be overly concerned about, but I want you to check into the hospital for some tests, and a laposcomptomy. That is where we put this tiny microscope down through your belly button and look around to see what is going on. Dr. Roe and I think you could possibly have a dermetoid cyst on one of your ovaries and this is best way to find out for sure. If that is what it is we will go ahead and do surgery and fix the problem. I don't want you to worry, you are in good health, and we just want to make sure everything is okay. I will have my nurse set everything up with the hospital and call you. If it is nothing you will only be in the hospital only two days." He rose from his seat and so did I. He then walked around his desk and put his arm around my shoulders and started to walk me towards the door. "Everything will be okay." His tone of voice was soft and reassuring, " Now you go home and talk to your husband and we will be in touch."

What an incredibly long drive home it was! I wanted to cry ... I did cry ... I couldn't imagine that this was really happening. By the time I got home I was in control again. Mike was already home, so I began to tell him what had happened at the doctors office and as I retold the story I began to weep, again. Mike simply took me in his arms and hugged me; he didn't say a thing, just held me tight. When I had finished he brushed away my tears and said, "Is that all?" "My whole life is flashing in front of my eyes. I am terrified of going to the hospital. I have only been in a hospital twice in my life ... once to be born and the other when I was eight and cracked my chin on the sidewalk and had to have three stitches at the ER. I just want it to all go away and pretend it is just a bad dream." When I said that Mike started to laugh at me which only made it worse, of course I had to retaliate and began to tickle him mercilessly. By the time we had both come back to our senses my next concern was no insurance to pay for any of this and we had just come back from Europe so our funds were short. Mike just said, "Don't worry it will all work out".

Two days later the doctor's office called with a date and a multitude of instructions to follow. I went to the hospital and got all the paper work taken care of, and learned what this little trip was going to cost us... that was scary. I was committed now, regardless of what I was feeling.

On August 19, 1979, with my husband by my side, we went to the hospital to begin what I was hoping would be a very short stay. I took my schoolbooks and my journal and as little hospital clothes as I could, praying that it would be just a couple of days. The smell of the hospital turned my stomach and I hated it before I had even spent anytime within its walls. After I am settled into my room the nurses started all their little routines, you know the ones where they keep coming back for blood and checking your blood pressure, sticking thermometers in your mouth … that type of thing. They were getting a little frustrated with me too because I wouldn't change into nightwear. I told them it was to early for bed and I did not have plans on taking up residence yet. Eventually Dr. Roe showed up and explained what kind of tests they would be performing the next day and assured me that he would see me tomorrow.

Shortly after Dr. Roe left, a nurse showed up with a really nasty tasting concoction that made me want to gag. Then she told me I couldn't have anything else to eat or drink the rest of the night. Needless to say, I wasn't happy about that. I didn't sleep well that first night. The medication they gave me hit early in the morning and the lady in the next bed was sick, so the nurses were in and out of our room all night long. Not to mention the unending blood samples needed to satisfy the vampires and the nurses' pleasant way of waking you from a sound moments sleep to see if you need a sleeping pill or shove a thermometer in your mouth. On top of the sleepless night when I finally did really doze off to sleep about 4 AM, the roused me at 6 AM to start getting me ready for tests that would start until 9 AM.

Mike showed up later that afternoon after work and I told him about all of the unpleasant tests that I had endured that morning. I had been poked with needles, given enemas that cramped me so bad that I had all but doubled me in half, had dye shot through my veins, had blood drawn where they had moved the needle and all done with good intentions. But I wanted to leave NOW! My husband couldn't understand why I was so upset. He tried to explain that they were just doing their jobs and I shouldn't let it get me so worked up. Mike sat on my bed and I buried my face in his shoulder while he tried to give me comfort. About 7:15 PM Mike had to leave for a previous appointment to work with the missionaries so I was alone … again.

Shortly after Mike left a nurse came in with another enema (that is the 3rd today) and it really hurt me. This was the final blow, or so I thought. I didn't feel sick when I came to the hospital yesterday, but boy I felt really bad now. All of a sudden the tears gushed down my cheek and I began to sob. I tried to call home to see if Mike was there yet and ask him to please come back, but to no avail. By the time my parents arrived I had worked myself up into quite a tizzy. Fortunately they snuck me up some real food, a fish sandwich, fries and a chocolate shake, which I was sure, was to be my last meal. As I told Mom what had happened I broke down and sobbed. She held me in her arms, just as she had when I was a little girl and cried with me. Daddy hugged us both and stroked my long hair. Then Daddy finally got a hold of Mike and told him, "You need to get over here right away and plan to stay the night." Before long Mike showed up and I grabbed on to him and hugged him like there wasn't going to be a tomorrow. My folks went home shortly after that. Mike couldn't understand why I was so upset and I couldn't explain it do him. All I knew was that I was scared to death of this whole ordeal.

A little while later a nurse comes in with a vaginal suppository. I told her no, I did not want it. I cried and hugged Mike even harder. He politely asked the nurse to come back in an hour. During that next hour Dr. Roe arrived with his clipboard full of papers. He shuffled through the papers and told me that they weren't exactly sure what it was, but I wasn't pregnant and that bloating could mean something else. He wanted to continue with the lapscomptomy but that they might need to do exploratory surgery depending on what they saw. I was mortified! He then proceeded to tell me all the things it might be from the least to the worst. When he mentioned cancer my heart skipped a beat even though he was fairly certain that that was not the case. He also explained the necessity of signing some sterilization papers, just in case the need should arise. But he didn't feel that would be the situation it was just a formality.

A lump formed in my throat and I tried to hold back the tears as anxiety welled in my chest and I began fearing the worst. Dr. Roe was very warm and caring as he told Mike and I what to expect over the next few hours and tomorrows turn in surgery. Mike just squeezed my hand as if to say, "don't worry everything will be okay."

Just a short time after Dr. Roe left a nurse arrived with the papers. My eyes still could believe the words that were at the top of the page ... Sterilization Form! Mike and I scanned over the form and then signed it, but in so doing I felt as if I just signed away my life and any hopes of my ever being a mother. I told Mike I didn't like the wording it sounded so ... so final.

Mike and I played some Rook and talked for a while to help take my mind off everything. I felt that I knew what was to happen tomorrow and my deepest fears of cancer burned in my soul. My Grandma Va had died of cancer when she was about 50, I didn't want to die, and I was to young and had too much life to live.

I was glad that Mike was there to comfort me. He just made me relax and feel peaceful with him there, he agreed to stay the night and I knew I would sleep easier. He kept saying, "don't worry everything will turn out okay." Soon I was beginning to get drowsy. I laid my head on the pillow and took his hand in mine and drifted off to sleep. But the sleep was fitful and the nurses were waking me up every couple of hours to take your temperature, blood pressure and more blood. I want to know who said you could get rest in a hospital ... they were lying!!

When I awoke the next morning I saw Mike sitting in the chair next to my bed and somehow it just made me feel better. . My parents arrived early to be with me for moral support. Then my husband and my father laid their hands on my head and gave me a blessing that promised that I would have a complete recovery. I put my faith in God and my family that everything would be all right, but the fear in my heart was still there. I was scared—No! I was terrified!!

The nurses came in and out all morning. I was supposed to go in for surgery at 9:30 a.m. so during this time I had to take a shower and put on that *ugly* hospital gown—you know the one that gives everyone a sneak peek as you walk down the hallway. Anyway I made Mike sit with me on the bed until it was time to go to surgery. Soon the nurses came in one after the other, one to take blood, one to take BP and temperature, one to give me a shot to make me sleep (they had to do it twice) and so on. Before long my mouth started to feel like cotton and they made me move to another bed and pulled up the sides. I felt barred in. But Mike stayed by my side and held my hand. I started to feel drowsy, but I didn't want to sleep yet, I made Mike give me a kiss before they wheeled me down the hall. I don't remember anything else until I got downstairs. I remember it being cold as I laid in the hallway and seeing Dr. Roe and Dr. Scholles. As they wheeled me into the operating room I remember everyone being dressed funny and the funny smells. The anesthesiologist put the IV in my hand and turned on the drip and said, "Now I want you to start counting backwards from 100." 100-99-98 and I was gone.

During the next several hours in surgery my doctors did what they do best; observe, consult, diagnose and treat. As time went by Dr. Roe had the unpleasant duty of calling my husband who was in the waiting room to tell him what their initial discovery. CANCER! Dr. Roe explained that they had sent one of ovaries and tubes over to the lab and were waiting for the test results to be sure. Thirty minutes later Dr. Roe calls back. Yes, it is definitely cancer. Not just any cancer, but a rare type of ovarian cancer in the beginning of its fourth stage.

I will never know the anguish my husband must of felt at that moment when he was called to make the decision about my future. *He* had to decide whether to leave everything just the way it was and hope for the best and treat it or for me to have a complete hysterectomy. Dr. Roe explained to Mike what he thought the best treatment was. I can't even imagine the pain and panic that gripped his soul as he gave permission for the sterilization that would save my life. It was more than just a hysterectomy, it also was scraping my whole insides in an attempt to make sure that they got all the possible growth associated with this type and stage of cancer.

After Mike hung up the phone he told my Mom what was going to happen and she gave him a big hug and they both cried. There were no words spoken, just tearful eyes and long pauses. Then Mike told Mom that he needed some time alone and he went outside to take a walk and think about what was about to happen and how it would affect our lives. My Mom went into the Chaplain's office and called my daddy, who had to teach a class that morning, and told him the outcome and wept.

Later when I began to wake up in the recovery room, I saw my mother's face and immediately asked where Mike was. She said that he had just gone down the hall to the bathroom and would be right back. I was so drowsy I don't remember much. When Mike arrived I made him give me a hug and a kiss and asked him to hold my hand. I remember being very sick to my stomach and vomiting until there was nothing left and having to hold my stomach and how much it hurt. I barely remember friends coming to see me later in the day or the flowers and balloons that began to arrive. I remember Daddy helping me on occasion when I was sick and my mother bathing my forehead. I slept most of the day. When the night came and it was time to go to sleep I gave Mike my blanket to keep him warm so he'd sleep better and the warmth of his hand in mine allowed me a certain peace of mind to drift of into a deep sleep.

The next morning I awoke and Mike was right there sitting in the chair, watching over me, just like my guardian angel. As I began to move and stretch a bit I became aware of just how stiff and sore I was. I couldn't move very well and the IV was still in my hand, but at least I wasn't nauseated any more and I was grateful for that. I recall that one doctor came into my room to check on me, yet nobody said anything to me about what had happened yesterday. After a while I turned to Mike and said, " Well is anyone going to tell me what happened, or am I going to have to guess?" Mike's face went blank, he took my hand and looked me in the eye and said, "They took everything, it was cancer." "No! No! " I cried, "It's not fair, I'm to young, my life is just beginning. It's not true, tell me it's not true!" Mike sat on the bed and held me tight and I just sobbed over and over, "this can't be happening, it's not true." His voice softened, "The doctors did everything they could. After they started the laproscope they immediately open you up and found that you had a growth on both ovaries. They took the one tube and ovary and sent it to the lab and called me and explained what was going on and said they'd try to save what they could. Thirty minutes later they told me they would have to take everything and that he was completely taken by surprise at what they had found. After the surgery Dr. Roe came down and talked to me and said that it had appeared to have started on the right ovary then jumped over to the left one and had begun to attach to the uterus. It was the shape of a cauliflower. It was a very rare type and unusual for someone as young as I was to have this type of cancer. He told me how very sorry he was that they couldn't save anything, but he did what he felt was best and he hoped they had gotten everything. Myn, he was really shocked by what he found, it was not what he had expected."

I could hardly believe my ears. I was numb. Yet in the furthermost reaches of my mind it suddenly dawned on me that Mike had been through a major trauma too. I didn't know how he felt as Dr. Roe told him what they had to do. All I knew at that moment was how hurt and crushed I was. I began my pity party all over again and I said through my tears over and over, "It's not fair, it's just not fair, what did I do to deserve this. I'll never be able to bear your children, never! Why me Lord? I've been good!" Mike never wavered he just sat there holding me and said, "I guess the Lord must have something very important for you to do or he wouldn't put you through such trials. He must know how strong you are. There are other children for us, just not now." I turned to him exasperated and said, "But what about now, will I never have a family? And if we adopt, they won't be yours. They won't be from my womb." "True, but they will still be ours," he said. Then with a touch of comedy he said, "Besides now you won't have to go through the pains of having babies or getting fat. Somebody else can do that for you." "I guess," I sighed, "but it's not the same. Besides will you still love me the same even though I'm gutted?" Mike simply laughed and kissed my forehead saying, "Yes! I love you now more than ever, and don't you worry our time will come. But right now I just want you to get better. I do really love you. Now I think you need to get some rest. Okay?"

I was totally exhausted after the mind blowing shock of what had occurred and I settled down and went to sleep knowing that my husband really did love me and that things could only get better from here.

Later on that afternoon, Dr. Roe came to my room to check on me. He inquired if I had been told what had happened. I told him that Mike had explained everything to me and I started to get teary-eyed, but tried hard to control myself. I knew that at this point that what had happened I couldn't change I was just going to have to accept it.

Dr. Roe then went on to say, "Tomorrow I would be given a form of radiation treatment, called radioactive phosphorus and he hoped that it would also be a deterrent from any further growth." He then told me to get some rest and he would check on me in the morning. A thin smile came to his face as if to say he was sorry for what had happened, and I knew he was and that he had done his very best for me.

The next morning Dr. Roe came by to see how I was doing and told me what to expect with today's treatment. Then he smiled and slipped out the door. A couple of hours later they came in with the radioactive materials, which they had to ship down from Oak Ridge. They tipped my bed so my feet were in the air and began to pump the radioactive phosphorous through a tube they had left in my stomach. Boy, was that stuff cold. Not only that but it made my stomach swell up like I was nine months pregnant (yeah, right). If that wasn't bad enough this stuff made me sick to my stomach. I couldn't keep anything down. I guess there are some ups to that, at least I didn't have to eat the hospital food.

For the next several days, I was a bad patient, with no patience. I hated being in the hospital. I hated what had happened to me. I hated that no one would accept that I had already accepted what had happened and I just wanted to get on with my life, and I really hated being sick. I begged my doctors to let me go home. I just knew I would get better faster if I could just go home. Of course they said, "no." I was healing rapidly and the doctors were happy with that, but there was no way they were letting me out of the hospital until I could keep some food on my stomach.

I decided that I wanted out, I felt trapped. My husband just laughed at me and said, "You need to be a good girl and quit giving everyone such a bad time." But I wanted out and would do whatever it took to get out of there including calling my mom and asking her to bring me a pot of her homemade potato soup. I just knew that it would make me feel better, it always had in the past. So the next day my mother shows up at the hospital with a large thermos of potato soup and boy was I grateful. I was getting really tired of popsicles, and that was the only thing I could keep on my stomach for several days. Needless to say I did manage to keep the soup down, but they still wouldn't let me go till they had removed my stitches, or should I say staples.

Finally, with the removal of my stitches they finally told me I could go home tomorrow if I was able to keep down my food the rest of the day. Even one day seemed good to me. Nine extremely long days in the hospital it seemed like an eternity to me. Most of the time I was alone and I bemoaned what I had seen as a tragedy in my young life. One day when my mom was there I asked the all famous line, "Why me God, I've been good. I've done everything I was supposed to do. Why are you punishing me?" Then just as soon as the word were out of my mouth I sat straight up and said, "Why not me? I'm young and strong and I can beat this!" Mom just smiled and said, "I know you can dear."

You know what? The more I accepted what I had been dealt, the more my friends would tell me I needed to face reality and quit dreaming. When I asked them why I should stop dreaming they would just try to remind me that I had just had major surgery and I needed to spend all my time concentrating on my recovery. I would say, "I'm fine. I just want to get on with my life." I didn't understand why it was so hard for them to believe that I had accepted or at least come to grips with what had happened to me. What was done was done! There was nothing I could do about it, except pray that God would bolster my soul and give me the strength to overcome what had happened and what was yet to come.

Going home was wonderful and I was so glad to be there. No nurses to poke you or wake you up in the middle of the night and my 6'1" teddy bear named Mike, to snuggle up with at night. I was really happy to be home.

The next few days proved to be difficult and yet profitable. I was determined that I was going to get on with my life in spite of how I felt physically and so I went to the university and applied for a job. Guess what? Two weeks after I got home from the hospital I had a full time job in the Office of Career Development at East Tennessee State University. The people there were great and they were willing to work with me, knowing that I would be taking chemotherapy treatments in the future. I needed to work to be able to get my mind off of my recent dilemma and this seemed to be just the ticket.

Over the next several weeks my emotions were as unbalanced as a super ball dropped off of a three-story building. They just bounced all over everywhere. One minute I would be ecstatically happy and the next I would be bawling my eyes out. My system was in shock from suddenly being thrown into menopause. A yo-yo had more fun than I did. Hot flashes, emotional ups and downs … totally unbalanced. On top of that my friends who were pregnant or who had babies avoided me like the plague. It was like I had a scarlet letter "C" branded on my forehead or something. They were so afraid that I couldn't cope or that they didn't know what to say to me that they just stayed away, except one friend, Cindy.

Cindy was younger than me by a couple of years and she was about six months pregnant. We had been friends since we were teenagers and she didn't want that to change. One day Cindy and her mother, Anne came over to check on me and see if they could do

It was late September now and I had been back and forth to the doctor several times since I left the hospital to follow my recovery. Dr. Roe couldn't believe how quickly I was healing and my positive attitude about all this. Now he was ready for me to go and see another type of doctor, a oncologist and begin some treatments to make sure that the cancer wasn't coming back. I wasn't to enthusiastic about this but I agreed to go and we set the appointment right then for the following week.

The time for my visit with the oncologist arrived and my husband and my mother both went with me for support and for the whole story. I remember being led back to a small darkish room where we all sat rather close to each other. I took Mike's hand and squeezed it tight; he was my support team. The doctor came in and introduced himself and then proceeded to thumb through my file. "Here is what we propose to do," he began in a very professional manner. "Because your cancer was advanced, your doctor and I have prescribed the most radical chemotherapy available. It involves three chemicals, one of them being liquid platinum which we will use to irradicate the cancerous cells that may be remaining within your system. You will need to take one treatment a month for the next year." I asked, "So what are the chances that this will work?" "There is about a 50/50 chance of success." Wonderful, I thought! Survive the surgery to be given only a 50% chance of success … yuck!

After that he proceeded to tell me all the downsides of the treatment, like you could suffer kidney and heart problems, lose your hearing, you will lose your hair after about the third treatment, etc. This was just a small list of all the things he mentioned.

It didn't sound very good to me and I wasn't at all convinced that this was the right thing to do. He continued to state that I would have to come in on a regular basis to have my blood checked to be sure that my blood count was high enough to be able to handle the treatment. Wait a minute, I thought, I have to be healthy in order for them to treat me, that seems odd! I guess I must of looked a little bewildered, because the next thing the doctor says is, " I know how you feel." "Whoa, wait just a minute," I thought. I then turned to him and said, "Oh really! Have you ever had chemotherapy yourself?" "No, I haven't", he said, "but, I have treated lots of people and can see how it affects them." At this point my dander was up and I was a wee bit irritated with this man. Mike tried to put us back on track by asking, "when will all this begin?" "Immediately," was the answer. "First we need to schedule an appointment to come in and have your blood drawn to check your blood count. If it is high enough we will schedule your first treatment." I could see that this confrontation was ending and I was glad. The doctor closes his book and says, "Your treatment will take about 6 hours by I.V. drip. It will make you nauseous. We have found marijuana works very well for lessening the effects of nausea. If you'd like I can give you a contact to get some before the treatment." My mouth hit the floor; "You've got to be kidding? I don't do drugs. You're a doctor, how could you even offer such a thing?" "Well truthfully, it doesn't matter if you smoke it or bake it in brownies as long as you get it into your system. It is however up to you." I flat out told him, "No, I don't think so." "It is your choice, but you should just think of it as medicine, not pot."

That was it! I had heard enough and wanted to leave, but the doctor left first. Mike just looked at me and said, "We needed to consider this carefully before you go jumping to any conclusions." I felt uneasy and confused about the chemotherapy and right then was not a good time to make that decision. The doctor made it sound like if I didn't have the treatments I would die and I didn't want that, but these treatments didn't sound right to me either. It was going to take a lot of prayer and research for me to make this decision. It was my life after all and I wanted to be sure.

I had learned a lot about cancer over the weeks since my surgery so I had the opportunity to make an informed decision now about this chemotherapy. I was stubborn. I never liked anyone telling me I had to do something for my own good. I wanted to make that decision on my own after some good old fashioned soul searching and studying. I was going to beat this thing called cancer and I was determined to do it my way and on my own terms!

Chapter Two

Healing the Body and Soul

Honestly, I didn't know where to start in my search for the truth. My father reminded me on more than one occasion that a great teacher once said, "I never said it would be easy. I only said it would be worth it." I relied on his faith and jumped into my studies of cancer and it's treatments with both feet.

I began by going to the local library to check out books on cancer. That led to books on nutrition. The first books I read were very vague on this subject but tended to lean towards the idea that there could be some link between cancer and nutrition, but that there had not been significant studies to verify this thesis. My bishop, at church, was a pediatric physician and very much into nutrition. When he heard of my studies, he provided me with much needed books on the subject.

Mike and I read every day about cancer and it's treatments, nutrition, diet, and the politics of cancer, anything we could get our hands on. We actually thirsted for the truth. At night we would sit and read and every so often one of us would find something we found interesting and had to read it out loud to the other person. Before long, Mike and I would have lengthy discussions about how we felt about what we were reading and how some of it could be implemented in our lives.

It absolutely amazed me at how much of cancer treatments were experimental. The majority of the treatments were still in the testing stages and since they didn't have anything else that worked any better, they continued its use. What we read was more like a horror novel than scientific research.

Most people don't have a clue as to what chemotherapy is or how it affects your body. To put it simply, the body is subjected to chemical poisoning and by doing this they hope to kill all the fast growing cells in your body. Needless to say that although cancer is a fast growing cell, it is not the only fast growing cells that our bodies manufacture; ie., skin, hair; nails, just to mention a few. Another thing this chemical dumping does to your body is destroy your immune system, so that while they are treating you for cancer you could get pneumonia and die because your body doesn't have what it takes to fight off the infection. The political part of all this is that when they list cause of death they will list that "died of pneumonia", not that they died of pneumonia caused by the cancer treatment they were receiving. And yet they conclude that cancer deaths are down, pretty ironic don't you think?

During the weeks of study we were doing I was still getting a call every week from the chemotherapist encouraging me to " get started with my treatments". I wracked my brain constantly about whether or not I should go ahead and have the treatments. I mean there was a 50 percent chance it would actually work, still I felt very uneasy about subjecting myself to more torture. The more we talked about it, the more agitated I became. Till finally I agreed to give it a try, mostly I think just to get them off my back.

The next week I went in and they did a blood check. I was still anemic so they couldn't schedule the first treatment. I was somewhat relieved at the prospect of having to wait a little longer. No sooner had that thought crossed my mind than the nurse came back with a big needle and said, "This is just a shot to boost your blood count". "What is it?" I asked. "It is testosterone. It will help build up your blood quickly. it has some possible side effects." " Oh, great," I thought. "Like what?" I asked. "You might notice dark facial hair and possibly your voice could be a little lower, but it will only be temporary." So I got my little shot and went home.

A week later I returned to the doctors' office to have my blood checked again. Guess what? Their little shot didn't work well enough so they were going to try it again. Only this time she comes back with a larger dose, how did she put it? Oh yes, "a double dose of testosterone … this should put hair on your chest," she chuckled. I didn't think that was very funny.

The following Sunday I took my place on the stand at church to lead the music for Sunday School and all was going well till I stood up to direct the first song. I raised my hand, and as I opened my mouth to sing nothing came out, not a squeak, not a note, nothing! I loved to sing, not just at church but also in musicals or even with the radio so when I could not even utter one note I was stunned. I was alright for the moment because I could lip sync the words but soon it was time for me to teach a new hymn to the congregation and I wasn't sure what I was going to do. I certainly couldn't sing the parts to help teach them the melody or harmonies, there was nothing there. So I opted for just having them listen to their parts as the pianist played them and acknowledging that my singing voice was swallowed by a "frog" and we would struggle through today. Luckily it was a simple hymn to learn and didn't require any vocalization on my part. I couldn't believe I couldn't sing not even one note. It didn't effect my speaking voice (all though my husband did tease me about my new husky voice), just my singing voice. What is strange is that it took me ten years to regain enough of my singing voice back before I could audition for any musicals. Guess what else? I went from a first soprano with a three-octave range to a bass. No kidding, I could sing the bass lines with ease, but couldn't even hit a C above middle C without cracking. It made me angry.

To add insult to injury when I went back to the doctors' office the next week, my blood was now normal and I could begin with my first treatment. Drats! I still was not convinced that this was the right thing to do, but I had agreed to at least have the first treatment and that kept them off my back about it. "Beep! Wrong Answer!"

The next day I went to the work and explained that I would be out of the office the following Thursday to begin my first treatment and not to expect me back in the office until the following Monday if all went well. They were very understanding and told me to take whatever time I needed, but just to come back well.

The month was now November and the weather outside had turned cold, the leaves had fallen from the trees and everything was gray and blustery. Just the type of weather you would expect for what I would come to describe as, "the worst mistake of my life." I arrived at the chemotherapists' office that Thursday morning with my mother because Mike had to work. I had eaten a light breakfast and had brought a book to read since they had told me that the treatment would last a couple of hours. I was in fairly good spirits and ready to face the challenge placed before me.

For Health's Sake

The nurse led me to a room with a chair and an exam table and not much else. She was fairly pleasant and explained that they would be placing an I.V. in my hand and that I would be receiving three different chemicals today as part of my treatment and that each would be followed by a saline solution to help wash it through my system. One of the chemicals would possibly make me nauseated and that if needed they could give me a shot to help with that. Mom was told that she would be in charge of me and that anything I needed just to take care of it. That of course was no problem for my mom, she had been taking care of me most of my life.

The first chemical they gave me was orange colored as I recall, but don't ask me what its' technical name was, I don't remember. It seemed to take forever for the first bag to drain, and I seemed to do okay with that one. Mom and I talked about different things and I even read a little bit. Then a bag of saline, I thought that was odd that the chemical was so bad that they needed to wash some of it out before they could give me the next chemical.

When the nurse came into put on the next chemical it was inside of a bag. I asked why. She said it was liquid platinum and that it was light sensitive. Oh, I thought that is what my wedding rings are made of, now my blood stream will be very rich for a while I joked with my mother. I was getting hungry and had brought something light to eat since they had told me I should have some type of food in my system during the treatment. So I ate an apple and a slice of cheese and drank some water. It wouldn't be too long before my body decided it did not like the newest chemical and I began to be sick to my stomach. At first it was just uncomfortable, but as time went by it got much worse.

When the time came for the third chemical I was holding my stomach and trying desperately not to vomit. The nurse finally asked if I wanted a shot to help with the nausea and I said I did. It amazed me that these medical people tried very hard not to be in the rooms where people were being treated and only checked in on you occasionally to see if you needed more drugs. The nurse soon returned and gave me the shot and within five minutes I was violently sick. As soon as I let up a little from emptying my guts, my mother went looking for the nurse and told her that she had better come back to the room and check on me that I was having some kind of reaction to the shot. Come to find out, not only did the chemo make me sick, but also I was having an allergic reaction to the anti-nausea medicine (my first allergy). My mother made sure that the nurse gave me something to help settle my stomach and also some rags to clean up the mess, since the nurses didn't do that. But this medicine did not help much either. It seemed like non-stop vomiting, a lot worse than with the radioactive phosphorous in the hospital. My head hurt, my sides hurt, my stomach hurt, and my throat hurt from all the dry heaves. My mother had to literally hold me up when my stomach convulsed, because my strength had completely drained away.

After six hours of grueling body torture, the last drug had been washed through my system with a saline solution and the nurse disconnected me from that blasted death tube. She told me I should take it easy and get some rest. I replied with a halfhearted laugh. The staff was so unfeeling about what it was really like to have gone through such an experience. They might, as well as placed me on a torture rack for six hours, I don't think it could have been any worse, it may even have been a relief.

Mom in the mean time went and pulled the van up to the back door so I wouldn't have to walk so far. She had to almost carry me to the van as I was little more than a wet, limp noodle by this time. As I slid into the van I caught a glimpse of myself in the side view mirror, my complexion was so white, I was even a little green. I told mom that I looked like I had just seen a ghost. She said, "no, you are one." I started to laugh when that urge to hurl came over me and mom handed me a lovely trash bag she had grabbed out of the room for just such an emergency.

We drove home in silence. I was so incredibly tired, it was all I could do to keep my head up. When we got to my house Mike was home and he carried me into the house and laid me on the couch where I stayed without moving the rest of the day. I sipped on ginger ale to soothe my stomach and moved as little as possible to avoid any further unforeseen upheavals. My head and body ached like I had been trampled by a herd of elephants; I had never felt worse in my 23 years of life, ever.

Existing on the couch somewhere between worse and worst, I swore I would NEVER, NEVER, NEVER let anyone put me through that again. There was nothing in this world that could persuade me that the treatment I had just gone through was good for my health. I always believed that God had created everything that we needed on this earth to help us solve our problems and now I was going to do what I believed.

Growing up I had been taught a code of health called the Word of Wisdom, which is found in *The Doctrine and Covenants*, Section 89. I decided that maybe there was something more in those words that I had missed and decided to prayerfully study its words again. I had always followed the basic principals of not drinking coffee, tea or alcohol, not doing drugs or smoking, but there was more to the code of health than that. Consider the following:

"…all wholesome herbs **[plants]** God hath ordained for the constitution, nature, and use of man—every herb **[plant]** in the season thereof, and every *fruit* in the season thereof; all these to be used with prudence and thanksgiving.

"Yea, *flesh* also of *beasts [animals]* and of the *fowls* of the air, … are to used *sparingly*; … they should *not be used only* in times of winter, or of cold, or famine.

"All *grain* is ordained for the use of man and of beasts, to be the *staff of life*, not only for man but for the beasts of the field and the fowls of heaven, and all wild animals that run or creep on earth; and these hath God made for the use of man only in times of famine and excess of hunger.

"*All grain* is good for the *food* of *man*; as also the *fruit* of the vine; that which yieldeth fruit, whether *in* the ground or *above* the ground—." (emphasis added)

I went to the dictionary to see how it defined some of these terms. It stated that the *Staff of life* is a "staple of diet." *Staple* is defined as "the sustaining or principal element; something used, needed, or enjoyed constantly" and *sparingly* means "barely, slightly, meagerly or sparsely." Suddenly my eyes were opened and I understood what I had been taught all my life. I had been following all these principals but not very closely. What my body needed now was stringent adherence to these simple guidelines. What I had gleaned from these few passages was that I should be eating mainly vegetables, herbs, fruits, grains; and meats sparingly. In later passages it promises that if you will live by these principals, "you will receive health in your navel and marrow in your bones, that you shall run and not be weary and walk and not faint." I thought about that, if you are eating properly you will be strong and healthy, it was perfectly logical.

As I continued to read, study, pray and contemplate the words before me, I came to the realization that not putting any harmful things into our bodies also included the poison that I called chemotherapy. Some people thought my decision to discontinue chemotherapy treatments were a bit rash, but then they were all blinded by the thought that I would die if I didn't have them. What most people failed to understand is I knew deep down in my soul that there was a better way to control my cancer. Sticking close to the principals of the Word of Wisdom was just one step towards returning myself back to complete health.

It didn't take much to convince Mike or my family that I was not going to take any more treatments. The hard part was convincing others that I had not lost my mind. I mean I was miserable for days after that initial treatment. I went back to work on Monday, but was so weak, that I didn't even make it the whole day. I was determined I was not going to let this get the best of me! I was going to fight feeling miserable with all my might! Trust me it was not easy, I felt really wiped out and for two days afterwards I couldn't eat because my stomach was still queasy. Gratefully, my family and the congregation of my church kept me in their prayers, because without their faith I think this would have been significantly worse.

The icing on the cake came a week after the treatment when the nurse from the chemotherapist office called and asked me to stop by the office after work. I said, "sure," just so I could give them a piece of my mind. When I arrived the nurse was all smiles and asked how I was doing. I replied politely, but the hair on the back of my neck was already rising. The nurse then held my chart and began to tell me that they had made a miscalculation on one of the drugs that they had given me, that they hadn't given me enough of the first drug. She then proceeded to look at a calendar and ask me what day would I like to schedule to come in and finish the treatment. My reply was quite swift and abrupt, I said, "How about the twelfth of Juvember?" She looked at me rather strangely like she didn't understand my response and I told her, "I will never come back!" "Why?" she asked. "If you need to ask why, you don't understand what your patients are going through with each treatment. Do you?" She looked dumbfounded and simply replied, "No" then in the next breath, "could you wait right here for a moment?" I nodded yes that I would, and she disappeared into the back office. The next thing I know the doctor appears and becons me to come back to his office. I know what he wants to do is convince me to continue for my own good. I simply told him I was not interested in being tongue lashed about the benefits I would receive from his treatments and that he could take his treatments and stick them where the sun don't shine. I was never going to subject my body to that kind of torture again. He began to interrupt me, but to no avail, I continued to tell him if he was only giving me a 50/50 chance of success I would take my 50 percent chance and run with it. I could win the battle without him or his poison. Before he had a chance to say anything else I turned and walked out the door.

I felt a big rush of exhilaration as I stepped outside of the office into the cool clean mountian air and got into my car. I knew I was doing the right thing for me. I also knew that there were a lot of people who would not agree with my radical decision to refuse further treatments. But I would show them all; that what I was about to do would work.

The next day I got a call from Dr. Roe about what had happened the previous day and he related his concerns about my decision and would I please reconsider. I told him politely that I appreciated his concern, but that I believed he had done what he thought was best for me at the hospital, and now I would do what I believed was best for me now. He accepted my decision grudgingly, but he did accept it. For the next several months however he and the chemotherapist would continue to try every way they could to get me to take some form of chemo. Their final attempt was for me to take a pill every day for the next 12 months, of course the side effects were that you would be nauseated 24 hours a day for 12 months. Does that sound good to you? It didn't sound good to me either.

Ten days after my first treatment I was finally feeling better and was working full time again. I have to say having a job to go to was good therapy for my mind. It gave me something to do besides feel sorry for myself. I did have 'pity parties' for myself on occasions and this day was going to be the first of several. I had gone outside to take my morning break and sat down on the curb to enjoy the beautiful crisp November day. As I was sitting there just breathing in the fresh air and watching the clouds I ran my hand through my hair to get it out of my face. As I brought my hand around to place it back in my lap I noticed that there was quite a bit of hair between my fingers. I thought, "No, this isn't happening, they told me I wouldn't lose my hair until after the third treatment." So I put my hand to the nape of my neck and grabbed a small handful of hair in an inconspicuous spot and pulled gently. What I got was a handful of hair. I was petrified; I couldn't believe it, so I did it again on the other side. The same thing happened. What was I going to do? How quickly was I going to lose it, would I lose it all or would it just get thinner? If I have to wear a wig, will people be able to tell that it is a wig?

I went back into work, but my mind was spinning out of control with this most recent discovery. The rest of the day went very slow and I couldn't wait to go home. When I got home from work that day my husband wasn't home yet, so I called my mother and told her what had happened. She wasn't too surprised, considering the previous week when Mike and I were over for Thanksgiving I complained that my hair hurt. In the meantime my husband had come home, I not only told him, but also showed him my latest dilemma. At first he gave me a hug and said it would be okay, then he started laughing and teasing me about being a female Kojack. Of course the only retaliation I had was to tickle him mercilessly. He of course finally gave in and told me he would still love my little baldhead. What a tease he was.

The next morning as I began to brush my hair, the brush would just fill up and I would have to clean my brush a couple times before I was done. It was pitiful. By the end of the week I had to wear wigs because there were literally just strands of hair here and there. I hated to look into the mirror in the morning. When I got home from work, I would throw the wigs on the bed and just scratch my head. The wigs were itchy. I couldn't stand to have my bare head hanging out. It made me feel very uncomfortable and ugly, so I would tie scarves around my head or wear a hat when I was at home. At night I always wore a scarf to bed even though my husband said it didn't bother him, it definitly bothered me!

Unbelievable as it may seem all this occurred within a two week time period of one treatment of chemotherapy. Try to imagine what was happening inside my body. The chemo was destroying every fast growing cell inside my body, what else was it destroying. It just burned my soul to think that the doctors office had the audacity to call me and want me to come in and have some more of one of those chemicals. What would have happened if they had given me a full dose to begin with? It made what I had read in *A World without Cancer* really come alive, what my body had just gone through was just short of chemical warfare. To top it off, chemotherapy was a big money racket, if you can imagine that one treatment cost over $850 in 1979 ... what does it cost today?

Along with the kickbacks from the chemotherapy I gained nearly 30 pounds. True most people who manage to continue with the treatments lose weight, but I didn't and the changes it put my system through have changed my metabolism in such a way, that it is now very difficult to take that weight off. Needless to say we don't stop trying either, but it is always a battle.

Nutritional Healing

Before I started the chemotherapy Mike and I had begun to make radical diet changes based on our reading. Hippocrates said, "Let your food be your medicine and your medicine be your food." Nutrition and health. It makes so much sense: "You are what you eat" and I will add what you do. What we did was sometimes challenging, but well worth the effort for me. Below are the changes we made:

1. *Milk.* This was the first to go. Man, was that one hard. When my parents moved out into the country there was a dairy farm down the road and my mom would go and buy fresh cows milk in large gallon jars with the cream still on it. You would let it set for a while and then skim the cream off the top. Oh, I loved a tall glass of ice-cold milk or a big bowl of ice cream for dessert every night (that was how I grew up). This was a very bad habit to break and I often craved milk, like some people need chocolate or cigarettes. It was hard. Why cut out milk? Milk is extremely hard to digest. I needed my body to put all of its efforts into healing not working double time so I could have that glass of milk. (See chapter 8 for more detailed information). After about a month of not drinking milk, just the thought of putting it in my mouth made me sick, and ice cream left a coating on the top of my mouth.

   We didn't include cultured dairy products like cheese or yogurt in our ban on milk, because the bacteria changes the way the body processes these items. Keep in mind though you still need to take care and use cultured dairy products in moderation.

2. *Meats.* Like all Americans I was raised to think that you had to have meat with every meal. Not so, as I was reminded in the Word of Wisdom, it should be eaten sparingly. We are not vegetarians. I still enjoy a good

piece of meat on occasion; the key here is *on occasion*. Meat has now become a side dish at our evening meal, not the main dish. When we first started this phase of our plan I could make a pound of hamburger last and entire week, still do. That is because I started using it as a flavoring agent in my casseroles, not the key ingredient. It is perfectly acceptable not to eat meat every day, even preferable. When you do decide to eat it, make sure that the portion is no bigger than your fist and remember that it takes more digestive enzymes to break it down. We found that if we were going to eat meat that evening that we always followed it with a digestive enzyme, like papaya, to help the body do its work.

3. *Sugars.* I was a classic junk food junkie. I loved fried pies, cakes, cookies, ice cream, candy bars or anything else sweet and gooey. It was the first thing I would look for when I got home from school and I didn't limit myself to just one. I was active and I figured I worked it off. Well in all my readings sugar was the number one bandit in the shoot-out. So I had to learn how to use less of it and start using more natural types. I started using fructose, date sugar, yellow D sugar and honey. Needless to say I did a lot of experimenting to create acceptable goodies. There is nothing wrong with a sweet treat occasionally. The key again is moderation, have a piece of cake but eat it slowly and enjoy it, don't inhale it and then need more because you didn't really savor the first one. If I have learned anything about sweeteners, it is your body doesn't care what kind it is, once it is in your system they all break down into carbohydrates. The biggest advantage to natural sweeteners is some of them provide some minerals and they have gone through less processing to leach out what little nutritional value they have (see chapter 10 for more information).

4. *Fruits and Vegetables.* We had always eaten them, but not in as great a volume as we did after we made the changes. Raw was good, when they were in season. Otherwise, we ate frozen vegetables and a few canned ones. Apples were number one on the hit parade, the whole apple so that I could benefit from the B-17 contained in the seeds. All fruits in their raw form were preferable, but sometimes I ate so much fruit I got tired of it. Variety is the key. Major benefit of fruits and vegetables besides all the vitamins and minerals are the energy and fiber you got from them (see chapters 4, 5 & 6 for more information). Join the Five-A-Day Club.

5. *Grains.* Like most people I used bleached white flour for everything, I didn't know any better. To get the biggest benefits from flour I changed to unbleached flour, whole-wheat flour, oat flour and some times soy flour. I experimented with different types of flours with various food products until I found what worked best. Grains go beyond flour though; we ate a lot more rice (white and brown), Couscous, oats, whole grain cereals, and other grains (see chapter 3 for more details on grains). Not only did this add more fiber to our diets, grains are packed with vitamins and minerals.

6. *Salt.* A big no-no. In our society the salt shaker comes standard on most kitchen tables. Why? Salt has been linked to a lot of health problems. Topping the pile is high blood pressure; I also add water retention to the list. You don't need to add salt; most vegetables come with enough sodium on their own that you shouldn't have to add more. What I found is that I

had to learn about herbs as seasonings to replace the need to use salt. Salt tends to mask the flavor, while herbs enhance the flavors of food. So keep the salt shaker on the stove for basic flavoring and off the table.

7. *Vitamins and Minerals.* I can't say enough about supplements when you are battling the Big C (cancer). For the **first year** after my surgery I megadosed on vitamins and minerals (after that I returned to quality multi-vitamins). I would not recommend this for everyone, but in my circumstance I truly believe that it benefited my quality of life. I can tell you that chemotherapy leaches out your energy and all the nutrients of value in your blood. Since it leaves you severely anemic, it is important to boost your system by taking high quality and quantities of supplements. What we did was to take a good natural multi-vitamin and then take additional tablets or capsules of vitamins that would benefit us the most. Sometimes it felt like that handful of vitamins was breakfast, there was so many of them. We increased our dosages on the following: A, C, E, B6,B12 and B15. We also included a papaya enzyme with each meal to aid in digestion or a papaya-based drink with the meal. It is amazing how much the enzyme can help if you are eating a meal high in protein.

8. *Fasting.* As strange as it may seem with all the food, vitamins and things in the environment that bombard our systems it does the body good to do without food for one day a month. While this is something that I have been doing most of my life for a spiritual reason I have found through study it is also good for the body. What happens is that it allows your body to eliminate toxins in your body and by doing this it renews your body. I also do this with my vitamins (no supplements on the weekends) to give my body a vacation. Think about it, when you return from a vacation you feel refreshed and rejuvenated. Fasting does the same thing for your body. Just remember when you eat after fasting make it simple, don't overdue it or you void the whole process.

Soul Snacks

You need to not only heal your body but you need to heal your soul. This may sound strange to you but when your body is ravaged by disease and you succumb to the medical world's treatments your spirit or soul also becomes damaged. You need to find a way to bolster your spirit and make it bright. Here are some hints I found helpful:

1. *Faith. Whether you are a religious person or not you need something to believe in. I found great solace in searching my scriptures for passages that would give me strength. I also attended church so that I could be with people who believed as I did and could give me both spiritual and mental support during this time of trial. It is a proven fact that people who believe in God have an 80-90% better chance of surviving a serious disease than those who don't have that conviction.*

2. *PMA (Positive Mental Attitude). PMA or positive mental attitude is imperative when you are dealing with cancer or any other life threatening diseases. You have got to believe deep down in your soul that you can and will overcome this trial. That this is just a step on the great ladder of life. You need to conjure up images of yourself free from the disease or condition that riddles*

your life. *I read in many books of how they were teaching children to draw a picture of what they thought their cancer looked like. Then picture in their mind, it being destroyed cell by cell. I believe that it works. You have to look in the mirror and say Yes, I Can and Yes, I Will Have a Good Day. I Deserve It, I'm Worth It. You have to believe it and you have to believe in yourself! Some people give themselves calendars or a book with positive affirmations. Do what it takes to think positively that you can deal with the trials and the healing ahead. Because you **CAN** do it!*

3. *Family and Friends. You can't do it by yourself. You can try and be some-what successful but what you need is someone who is willing to* **listen** *to your crying, whining, complaining and your successes. Not a therapist, just someone who cares about you and someone you can rely on to be there when you need them. My best friend is my husband. No matter what the problem or my complaint he was always there for me. I don't think that my success would have been as wonderful or as sweet without him there to cheer me on. Family and friends are good cheerleaders, have a bunch!*

4. *Get Educated. Knowledge is power. Read books on both conventional, toxic-based cancer treatments, and on nontoxic cancer treatments. The more you know about your options, the more likely you are to make the right choice. Never be afraid to ask questions. I would not have been able to make the decision to can the whole chemotherapy gig if I hadn't done my homework. Without books, and today without the worldwide web you can starve your mind of the chance to gain knowledge and weigh out both sides of the issue before you make a decision. It is a wonderful feeling to find out that your gut feelings are more than just that. My research lead me to realize that even in an era that was just beginning to find the connection between nutrition and cancer that my gut feelings were right. I have followed that same feeling now since 1979 and look where I am today. Healthy and Happy.*

5. *Service. Get lost in helping others, because in so doing you are helping yourself. It can be anything; helping at a soup kitchen, playing a game with a child, making quilts for the homeless, working with the handicapped, being a good listener, taking a plate of cookies to a new neighbor, the choices are endless. Through serving in even the smallest way your burden is lightened as you give of yourself. The joy is in the giving … give often.*

6. *Keep a Journal. Sometimes you get really frustrated and you don't want to talk about what is bugging you, so write it down. Writing is a great way to relieve stress and cleanse your soul. By putting it on paper you not only keep a record of what is happening in your life but it also helps you work through your problems. So go ahead rant and rave, cry, get all out of your system via the pen and you will feel better.*

My journey through the world of cancer and its treatment was hard on my family and me. I was a determined and often a very angry young woman that first year. What I learned I wanted to share with others. I know that you must feed your soul and you must nourish your body, and if you will do that you will be a winner. The choices I made, made me a stronger person and have given me the opportunity to pass on to others what I have learned. Would I have made a different choice today? No! I stand fast on the knowledge that what I did made a difference.

Today's medical research confirms that there is a link between cancer and nutrition. Everyday I read in the newspaper, magazines or on the Internet that they are finding new evidence that we are what we eat and what we eat makes a difference. The American Cancer Society predicted that a full third of the 563,000 cancer deaths in 1999 will be nutrition-related. The American Institute of Cancer Research recently put out a single comprehensive report, "Food, Nutrition and the Prevention of Cancer: A Global Perspective." What is their bottom line? "Cancer is a preventable disease."

I have written this book *For Health's Sake* in an effort to give you a stepping stone to knowledge along with some recipes to start you on your way to a healthier lifestyle. There is no magic in what I have done and I am no hero. I am someone like you who went searching for the truth and I thank God daily, that He was looking out for me and showed me where to *look* for the answers. I now pass on to you what I have learned. I am still learning. I am an ever-conscious student of nutrition and life and that is why I have revised this book after 18 years. I hope you will use this book in good health. If I've peaked your interest in nutrition, take the next step and study some more. I have listed a few of my favorite books and websites in the back of the book. Don't be afraid of knowledge, it can be a great journey!

Wishing you Love and Good Health,

Mylinda Butterworth

Healing Body and Soul

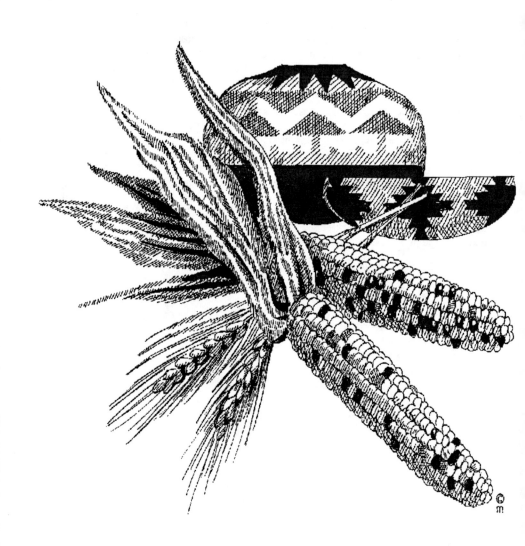

Chapter Three

Wheat and Other Grains of Knowledge

You've heard about wheat and corn, barley and soy, but what do you really know about grains? Probably not more than their names, there are __ types of grains in the world each with its own nutritional properties. Grains have nourished the world for several millennia. It is time to rediscover grains and all their great attributes. Grains are high in complex carbohydrates, fiber, vitamins, minerals and protein, and low in fat, grains form the base of the food pyramid. So why is it that we tend to neglect grains as a whole food and only see it as a slice of bread for a sandwich? The following is a list of the assorted grains as well as several nongrains, which can add to your platter taste and diversity.

Amaranth - A tiny mustard-colored seed about the size of a poppy seed with a nutty almost peppery flavor; not a true grain. Available as seeds and flour.

Barley - A true grain with nutty flavor and a slightly chewy texture. Available hulled, or as flakes, pearls or pot (Scotch).

Buckwheat - These triangular granules have a strong, distinctive nutlike flavor that marries well with earthy and hearty foods. Not a true grain but the fruit of a leafy plant belonging to the same family as sorrel and rhubarb. Forms of Buckwheat; Buckwheat groats are whole crushed kernels that have had its hard outer shell removed. Kasha is roasted buckwheat groats. Buckwheat flour contains about 7 percent of the hull and is gluten free.

Corn - A yellow, white, red, or blue kernel that can be eaten, fresh, dried, cracked, or ground into a variety of products. Originally the generic term for any grain in Europe. *Forms of Corn:* Cornmeal is ground dried corn and is available in yellow, white, red or blue grain. Grits are corn that is cracked into very small pieces. Hominy is corn that is soaked in limewater to remove the hull, then dried.

Kamut - Ancient variety of wheat. Available as berries, flour, grits and pasta.

Millet - Tiny, round, shiny, pale yellow to reddish orange seeds that have a bland flavor. Because it's gluten-free, it is usually tolerated by those allergic to wheat. Available whole, cracked and ground. *Forms of Millet:* Couscous of North Africa is cracked millet that has been steamed. Millet meal if finely ground and used for baking. Millet flour is more finely ground. Puffed millet is made from the whole grain heated under pressure.

Oats - Available as bran, groats, rolled, or steel-cut (Irish). Forms of Oats: Groats are whole crushed kernels that have not been milled, polished, or heat-treated. Grinding the groats makes oat flour. Old fashioned rolled oats

Quinoa - Pronounced keen'-wah; tiny ivory-colored, flat-oval seeds about the size of millet that have a delicate flavor. Not a true grain but the fruit of a leafy plant belonging to the same family as spinach. Available as whole seed, flour and pasta.

Rice - Types include long, medium and short grain and regular and aromatic. Available as whole, instant, grits, meal and flour. *Forms of Rice:* Brown rice is the whole unpolished rice grain, with only the outer hull and a small portion of the bran removed. Rice flour is finely milled rice, and is sometimes combined with wheat flour.

Rye - Similar in appearance and closely related to wheat but contains less gluten. Available cracked and as flakes, grits, berries, and flour. *Forms of Rye*: Rye Flakes are the rye equivalent of rolled oats. Rye Flour is ground rye. Light and medium rye flour are then sifted which removes much of the bran. Dark rye flour is what is generally used to make pumpernickel bread.

Spelt - Ancient variety of wheat. Available as berries, flour and pasta.

Sorghum - is believed to have originated in Africa where it was domesticated. It is a major food grain in Africa and India but virtually unknown in America except as cattle feed or syrup. *Forms of Sorghum*: Outside of the U.S. it is roasted and eaten like popcorn, milled and cooked into porridge or mush and ground into flour to bake flat bread.

Teff - The tiniest grain. It has a light, nutty flavor.

Triticale: Pronounced tri-ti-kay'lee. The nutritious hybrid of wheat and rye, it contains more protein than wheat, although less converts to gluten when it's used in baking. Available as berries, flakes and flour.

Wheat - One of the oldest cultivated grains, known in ancient times as the staff of life. Available as berries, bulgur, cracked, grits, flakes, and flour. *Forms of wheat*: Couscous is finely cracked wheat. Wheat Germ is just what its name implies; the vitamin and mineral-rich wheat embryo that is separated out when flour is refined. Bran Flakes is sometimes called unprocessed bran. Bulgur or cracked wheat. Semolina is the coarse granular meal from the endosperm of durum wheat and is generally used to make pasta. Graham flour is whole-wheat flour in which the starchy part of the wheat kernel is finely ground but the bran is left coarse and flaky. Whole-wheat flour is less coarse than the stone-ground variety and may contain flour additives like malted barley flour. Whole-wheat pastry flour is made from soft whole wheat that is finely milled. All-purpose flour is refined white flour, which is a blend of hard and soft wheat flours. It is chemically bleached, and then enriched with the addition of iron, niacin, thiamin and riboflavin. Unbleached flour is unbleached white flour. It is ground from the endosperm of the wheat berry (it does not contain the germ or the bran) and is not treated with chemical bleaching

Wild rice - The grain of an aquatic grass native to North America; not a true rice.

The U.S. Department of Health and Human Services, the National Cancer Institute, the American Heart Association, and many other health organizations, and the Surgeon General concur that we should reduce the amount of fat and calories and increase the amount of fiber and complex carbohydrates in our diets. Grains are low in fat and calories, high in fiber, and one of the best sources for complex carbohydrates. They are also a cholesterol-free protein source - 1 cup generally provides less than 2 grams of fat, no cholesterol, and from 120 to 280 calories. Current guidelines advise that grains and other complex carbohydrates should supply more than 50 percent of the calories you consume.

Chapter Four

Fresh and Fruity

J ust imagine a big bowl of fruit salad, with mouth-watering strawberries, juicy peaches, "dribble-down your chin watermelon," ... well you get the picture. Very few people can resist the smell or the luscious taste sensations that you can get from fruit. Adam couldn't resist the apple proffered by Eve and they covered themselves with the leaves from a fig tree. Not only has fruit been a tempter in history, but also it was a highly valued commodity.

Today our perception of fruits and vegetables in our diets is low on the proverbial totem pole. But the consumption of fruits and vegetables is widely believed to have multiple health benefits including lower risk for many cancers, diabetes, stroke, and now coronary heart disease. A recent study published by Eric Rimm, of the Harvard School of Public Health in Boston, MA, concluded that higher intake of folate and vitamin B6 -found in many vegetables and fruits - is associated with substantially reduced risk of heart attack and coronary heart disease in women.

With so much overwhelming evidence of the relationship between fruit and vegetable consumption and cancer, along with the fact that most of Americans only eat 3.4 servings per day, (five per day being the recommended amount) caused some concern to the National Cancer Institute. The National Cancer Institute then joined with the Produce for Better Health foundation and launched the *Five A Day for Better Health* program in 1991. Their whole mission has been to encourage Americans to eat five or more servings of vegetables and fruit every day.

My children have their favorites. My daughter likes me to core the middle of an apple and stuff it with peanut butter, my son like peaches, my husband is a whole apple (core and all) a day man, mom loves apricots and me? Well I like them all. Fruits are so sweet and tasty, how can you resist? With over 300 varieties of fruits and vegetables available, we shouldn't get bored because there is bound to be something everyone likes

Fruits and vegetables are good for you. We all know that they are. Not only do they provide essential vitamins and minerals, but they also provide us with a powerhouse of energy. Our lives are so busy, simply having fruits and vegetables available and accessible, helps increase the likelihood that they'll get eaten. Fruit is the original snack food. With that in mind, I have listed just a few of the types of snack foods you can get in your local grocery store and some of their qualities.

Apples supply two types of fiber that are linked to good health. Insoluble fiber, found in the skin of the apple, keeps your intestinal tract healthy and helps prevent certain types of cancer. Soluble fiber helps to keep blood sugar steady, make you feel full, and reduce your risk of heart disease by pulling cholesterol out of your body. Apples also contain phytochemicals (plant chemicals) called flavonoids that also may lower heart disease risk by helping keep artery-clogging plaque from forming. Quite a health package for only 80 calories in a medium-size apple!

Cranberries are a terrific nutrition package. One cup of cranberries — two

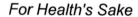

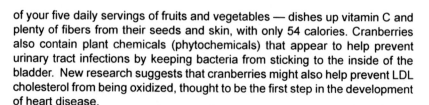

of your five daily servings of fruits and vegetables — dishes up vitamin C and plenty of fibers from their seeds and skin, with only 54 calories. Cranberries also contain plant chemicals (phytochemicals) that appear to help prevent urinary tract infections by keeping bacteria from sticking to the inside of the bladder. New research suggests that cranberries might also help prevent LDL cholesterol from being oxidized, thought to be the first step in the development of heart disease.

A cup of grapes — that's two servings toward your five daily servings of fruits and vegetables — supplies about 60 calories and vitamin C. Grapes also are loaded with phytochemicals (naturally occurring plant chemicals) with fancy names like quercetin, reservatrol, anthocyanin and catechin. These phytochemicals work as antioxidants that protect cells from damage and are thought to reduce cancer risk.

The first letter in citrus is a clue to the nutrient that citrus is best known for-vitamin C. A single serving of citrus - one orange, half of a grapefruit, two tangerines or six ounces orange juice- easily fulfills the daily requirement for vitamin C. But that's not all. Citrus fruits, in particular oranges, also supply the B vitamin folate and vitamin B6, which have been shown to reduce heart disease risk. A recent study in the Journal of the American Medical Association found that women who consumed the most folate and vitamin B6 had the lowest incidence of heart disease. Citrus also have antioxidants that appear to protect cells in the body from cancer-related changes. All of this in a convenient, versatile and easy-to-eat package.

Blue foods have a special appeal with kids — and blueberries are one of the few naturally blue foods. This anthocyanin (a flavonoid or plant antioxidant), together with fiber, folic acid, vitamins A and C, carotenoids, ellagic acid, only a few calories, and other antioxidants, make blueberries a powerhouse in reducing the risk of cancer and heart disease.

It's hard to imagine better an example of packaging than a banana! Bananas are easily digested, and are high in nutrients like potassium and vitamin B6, a vitamin that may help reduce heart disease risk. Bananas are even sources of vitamin C. and depending on the size, a banana counts as up to two of your five-a-day servings of fruits and vegetables.

Peaches and nectarines look and taste alike, sharing a common nutrition profile. Each is a good source of vitamin C and has only 40 calories in a medium-sized fruit. Their orange color means that they also supply beta-carotene, an orange plant pigment that may have cancer-preventing and other health benefits. Plums, like most of their fruity cousins, are virtually fat-free and dish up vitamin C. These stone fruits, along with kiwi fruit, are good sources of vitamin C. A medium kiwi supplies more than the daily recommendation for vitamin C, along with folate, several antioxidants and phytochemicals that protect your body's cells from damage. Plus, pears have more fiber than almost any other fruit.

Did you know that the average strawberry has over 200 seeds? These crunchy seeds give strawberries much of their fiber. And that's not all. Strawberries also supply vitamin C and folate, a B vitamin that plays a role in preventing birth defects and protecting against heart disease.

Now that you now the value of fruits in your diet do you want to know a shortcut to measuring a serving size? Generally, a fruit and vegetable serving is about the size of your fist. A serving of leafy greens should be larger than your fist, while a serving of dried fruit is smaller than your fist.

Fruits and vegetables provide so many benefits. Not only do they taste and look great, but research has shown that those who eat five or more servings of fruits and vegetables every day have half the risk of developing cancer as those who eat only one or two servings a day. Fruits and vegetables are also important in reducing the risk of heart disease, stroke, obesity, and for just downright feeling good.

It is really easy to add more fruits to our diet and once you get started you'll wonder what the fuss was all about. Follow some of these tips they will become second nature to you. Before long you will be a member of the Five- A-Day club.

- Top off a bowl of cereal with a smiling face from sliced bananas for eyes, raisins for a nose, and an orange slice for a mouth.
- Drink 100% fruit juice in easy-to-tote boxes or cans.
- Pack ready-to-eat fruits and vegetables for a convenient snack on the go.
- Add fresh fruit and vegetables to foods you already eat - like berries and bananas to yogurt and cereal; vegetables to pasta and pizza; and lettuce, tomato and onion to sandwiches.
- Keep fruits and vegetables visible and easily accessible. For instance, store cut and cleaned produce at eye-level in the refrigerator.
- Make a quick smoothie in the blender by pureeing peaches and/or nectarines, a touch of your favorite fruit juice, crushed ice, and a light sprinkling of nutmeg.
- Keep a big bowl of ripe summer fruit on the table for passers-by to pick up on their way out.
- When watermelon is in season, cut off a section and cube it. Put it in a bowl in the refrigerator so it is easy to eat. It is also good cubed and frozen.
- Toss grapefruit and/or orange sections in a fresh crunchy salad of mixed greens - the sweet citrus and crisp lettuce are an incredible wake-up call for the taste buds, and the juice from the segments moistens each leaf.
- Eat dried fruit instead of candy.
- Make frozen fruit kabobs for kids using pineapple chunks, bananas, grapes and berries.
- Go shopping with your children and let them pick out a new fruit and vegetable to try.
- Buy ready-to-eat packaged fresh vegetables that are already cleaned.
- Add broccoli or cauliflower florets; bell pepper strips, peas or squash to your next pasta dinner and voíla - pasta primavera! One-half cup of cooked or canned vegetables makes one of the five-a-day serving recommendations.
- One of the easiest ways to add vitamin C to your diet is to drink a glass of orange or grapefruit juice on your way to the office or with breakfast, lunch or dinner.
- Perk up deli salads like coleslaw, chicken, or tuna with apple chunks, pineapple, or raisins.

- Use fruit as toppings for pudding or yogurt; fresh raspberries, blueberries, strawberries, peaches and dried fruits add sweetness without the fat. Or, blend fresh fruit into a smoothie with yogurt and ice.
- For an easy make-ahead side salad that will last all week, mix tomato, cucumber and onion slices with vinegar, salt and pepper and sprinkle with a few drops of olive oil.
- You don't have to skimp on taste to find desserts that are good for you. Baked apples are so easy to make that your kids can help prepare them. Simply core an apple without cutting all the way through, fill with raisins or marshmallows, sprinkle with cinnamon and sugar and microwave or bake until soft. One apple packs 4.5 grams of fiber. Bake bananas until black, slice open and sprinkle with brown sugar to yield a delicious custard-like treat, too.

Now that you have some ideas on how to add fruits to your diet (that was easy wasn't it?) you really ought to know how to store them.

Fresh fruits in season are your best nutritional bet. The key here is in season, we don't know how long these fruits have been in storage since they were picked and the longer they sit around the more nutrients are lost. So when the season is gone buy frozen fruit first because they retain more of the nutrients than canned and generally have less added sugars. Check the label before you buy.

In general buy fresh produce that has been ripened on the plant. Avoid, wilted or shriveled-looking produce as well as produce with bruises or spoiled spots. Buy more than you'll be able to use in the next few days. If you can't shop often, from a nutritional perspective you will be better off buying frozen fruits. That is something that the Europeans still have over us is their open market place where you can go daily and buy fresh produce. Of course, here if you are lucky enough to find a farmers market you will also have the ability to buy it fresh in season.

Whether fresh, frozen, or canned, all foods lose vitamins and minerals during storage. To minimize losses, keep canned foods at about 65° F or cooler, and maintain frozen foods at 0° or below. Try to use frozen produce within a couple of months, certainly within 6 to eight months to maintain quality as well as nutrients. There is nothing more disappointing than to take out a bag of fruit from the freezer, that is ancient, and to take a bite into tasteless mush. So use a permanent marker and write the date on the outside of the bag to make sure that it is used before it is unusable.

As for fresh fruits take a tip from the supermarkets, are they in a cooler section or are they left out at room temperature. True some of us prefer our oranges cold, but they are juicer and less likely to be woody if left out in a bowl. Not to mention, they will get eaten faster if left out in plain site. It is okay to refrigerate all your fruits (bananas skin will go black but it slows down aging), just don't forget that they are in there or you begin to find mummified fruit hiding on the shelves.

Remember that we all need to eat five *or more* servings of fruits or vegetables every day for better health. An ounce of prevention today truly is worth a pound of cure tomorrow!

Chapter Five

Veggie Power

S it up! Don't slouch! Eat your veggies!" Didn't your mother tell you the same things as mine did? Of course she did! When we were babies and just learning to eat solid foods our parents would play all sorts of games to get us to eat our vegetables. You know like, "Open wide here comes the airplane." We were all encouraged to eat our vegetables so that we would grow up to be big and strong. We fantasized that we would be as strong as Popeye if we ate our spinach. Let us not forget one other thing most parents did ... the guilt trip, "You eat those vegetables, don't you know that there are starving children in China who would love to have what is on your plate?" My brothers comment was always, "Where's a box and I'll ship it to them?" In spite of all the things we did or didn't do to get our kids to eat vegetables, today's kids only like them if they are fried or smothered in sauces or butter. "What's a Mom to do?"

The best thing you can do is to introduce vegetables early in a child's diet. Sure you give them that tasteless paste when they have no teeth, but you can do them a bigger favor by giving them the real stuff. By that I mean as soon as you can give them fresh vegetables. As soon as my daughter was able I did that with her and don't you know that by age three she was eating green peppers like they were apples and preferred them to a cookie. It can happen, sure she likes cookies like any other child her age, but her preference runs to the fresh fruits and vegetables she can find in my refrigerator or in the garden. How do you get them to eat them? Make them easily available. When my daughter Nicole was very young she always wanted to get into the refrigerator and she was always hungry. So one day I simply made the bottom shelf in the fridge hers and filled it with all sorts of freshly washed fruits and vegetables. Then when she was hungry she knew where she could go to get something to eat. If you make good food readily available to a child they will grow up loving what tastes good and is good for them. Adults are no different. If when you come home from the store you take a few minutes to fix up a bowl of cut celery, carrots, radishes or have a drawer full of apples, plums, grapes or whatever is in season ready to eat ... they will eat. We live in a fast food society. When we are hungry we want to eat, and we want to eat it now! There is nothing so perfect as fruits and vegetables for quick pick a fast snack or me up. Think about it, what other food do you know that comes in its own packaging?

What is our problem with fruits and vegetables in our diets? Is it that they're boring? Yes, sometimes I think that is true. When you fix vegetables for your meals do they just lie there on your plate looking plain and boring? Probably. Then fix it! It is so easy and your tastebuds will thank you. What is the fix you say ... herbs. Yes those delightful, sweet, savory, wonderful herbs. OK, I know that it sounds to easy but contemplate this ... your faced with a bowl of corn, it is a pretty color and goes very well with the other items on the plate but it is boring. What do you do? You open up the cupboard door, which is filled with all those delightful herbs and spices, and you start sprinkling on the parsley or the dill or the rosemary and you mix it well and bingo you have just given your tastebuds a new tantalizing flavor buzz. Easy wasn't it. This is one of those things that you have to just jump in with both feet, because truthfully most of don't have a clue on how to use herbs to enhance the flavor of our foods. If you are willing to try it just a few times, believe me you will be hooked.

Now here is some big news ... vegetables have staying power! Yes, we can derive the same amount of energy from vegetables as we can from meat and it requires our bodies to do substantially less work to do it. Know something else? Vegetables are not only delicious and easy to serve but, they are also some of the most nutritionally sound foods we can consume, chock-full of vitamins, minerals and other nutrients we need to maintain good health. Funny thing is it took the scientific society years and years to finally realize that something as simple as "eating your veggies" can be helpful in fighting diseases like cancer and cardiovascular disease just to mention a few,

Vegetables can be broken down into seven different types; leafy greens, stems, roots and tubers, vegetable flowers and flowering vegetables. Below I will give a brief description of each different family of vegetables.

Leafy Greens: Cabbage, Lettuce, Chard, Spinach, Collards, Watercress, Kale, Dandelion, Mustard and Turnip Greens. These are probably the richest in nutrients of any foods in the vegetable kingdom. They are high in vitamins A and C and the minerals magnesium, potassium and iron. Calcium is also very high in the greens. Did you know that there is twice as much calcium in a cup of spinach as a cup of milk.

Stems: Asparagus, Leeks, Celery, and Rhubarb. This category is basically what is left over after the roots, leaves and flowers. Leeks are probably more similar to the bulb or root group, while asparagus is in a world of its won. Most of these plants are low in calories and very good in fiber content. Good sources of A and C.

Roots and Tubers: Beets, Parsnips, Carrots, Rutabagas, Garlic Turnips, Onions, Radishes, Potatoes, Sweet Potatoes and Yams. The root vegetables (those that grow underground) also include the tubers (potatoes) and bulbs (garlic and onion) are probably the most commonly consumed group of vegetables throughout the world. One of these root vegetables might be cooked along with the main dish or as a dish itself, as part of a mixed vegetable dish, or as a seasoning for other dishes. Potatoes, carrots and garlic and onion are the most popular. These vegetables vary in their nutrient content, though they all are "starchy"; that is, contain a high portion of complex carbohydrates. Carrots and sweet potatoes are both very high in beta-carotene, which generates vitamin A. Cooking potatoes, are high in vitamin C and lots of other nutrients. Most of these root vegetables, especially yams, are rich in potassium.

Vegetable Flowers: Artichokes, Brussels Sprouts, Broccoli, and Cauliflower. Vegetable flowers are actually the early part of the potential flower of the plant, picked and eaten before they progress into a "real" flower. These vegetables tend to be low in calories and high in carbohydrates but also have some protein and good fiber content. They are all good in vitamin C, folic acid, and potassium, and broccoli is very rich in vitamin A. Artichokes are actually the flower of a thistle plant that is very beautiful when left to fully flower, while cauliflower and broccoli are members of the highly nutritious cruciferous family, thought to help reduce the incidence of cancer.

Flowering Vegetables: Cucumbers, Pumpkins, Eggplants, Squashes, Peppers and Tomatoes (even though some folks still say a tomato is a fruit). These plants are many, mainly growing on small bushes and vines. Each one has many different varieties. The flowering vegetables are botanically like fruits in that they carry the plant's matured seeds for the next generation. These vegetables grow after and in replacement of the flowers, much like a citrus tree. And some, such as tomatoes and cucumbers, are as juicy and nutritious as many fruits. Squashes are multiple and vary from small, soft, high water content zucchini and summer squash to hard, starchy drier ones, such as acorn and hubbard squash. Even the pumpkin is in the squash family. These vegetables are prevalent in minerals such as phosphorous, silicon, iron, magnesium, and calcium. Many are sources of vitamin A, C, niacin and potassium.

Ocean Vegetables- Seaweed: Agar-agar, Kelp, Arame, Kombu, Dulse, Nori, Hijiki, and Wakame. The vegetables that come from the sea are some of the most nutrient-rich foods we have, particularly in iodine, calcium, potassium, and iron, and some being very high in protein as well. Since these plants are constantly bathed in the mineral-rich ocean waters, they have a regular supply of nutrients. Sodium, however, can also be concentrated in these saltwater vegetables that supply food for many fishes. Most seaweed contain algin, a fiber molecule that binds minerals. When taken into our body, it can attract various metals within our digestive tract, possibly including heavy metals such as lead and mercury, and take them out of our system. It is further wise to include sea vegetables in our diets more regularly to provide good mineral nutrition and reduce possible absorption and utilization of similar radioactive compounds, such as iodine 131, from environmental or medical sources.

Legumes-Peas and Beans: The legume vegetables are a special class of the pea and bean plants, which contain edible seeds inside pods that grow after the plant flowers (For detailed information on legumes read chapter 6). The legumes are an interesting food, mainly a mixture of protein and starch, with many positive qualities as a food. They are low in calories, low in fat, a good complex carbohydrate, and fairly high in fiber, which may help intestinal action and even help to reduce cholesterol levels. Most important, though, especially for the vegetarian, the legumes are a good and inexpensive protein source. They cost on the average about 3 per pound of protein, whereas egg protein may cost about 6 and meat protein more like 12 per pound. And the extra advantage is that the beans have less than 10 percent fat content. So, though beans may be considered the poor people's meat, they might better be known as the healthy people's meat.

Vegetables can be a veritable smorgasbord of flavors if they are prepared well. Cooking your vegetables not only softens their tough outer skins but it renders them more digestible, so that, in turn, we can assimilate them completely and benefit fully from their nourishment. Some people think that the only way to fix fresh vegetables is to boil or steam them. not so. Microwaves are great because they require a shorter cooking time, thus leaving more vitamins. Let's not forget other methods of preparation like stewing and braising, broiling or grilling, sautéing, baking or roasting and even pickling. Bet you never thought there were so many ways to cook your vegetables. Cooking times for vegetables, even in the best recipes, are only estimates, since everything hinges on how you cut them as well as the size and freshness of the vegetables. When are they done? Most cooks consider a vegetable done when you can easily pierce it with a fork or when you taste it and it is the tenderness you like.

Next big question ... canned versus frozen, that is a big issue for a lot of people. My preference for most vegetables is frozen because they taste more like their fresh counterpart, but the truth is, unless they are cooked to death your canned vegetables retain almost the same nutritive value as the frozen vegetables. This is really is a preference call. When at all possible start with fresh vegetables that are in season for the most flavor and vitamins.

Just one last thing if you want the power of veggies to be a big part of your life start thinking of them as the main dish and your meat as the side dish. You will find that not only are you cutting a large amount of fat out of your diet, but that you actually have more energy after a meal. That big slab of meat on your plate (even if does taste good) can cause you to feel sluggish and actually make you feel groggy after the meal. So get pumped on vegetables and make your mother (and yourself) proud by eating all your vegetables.

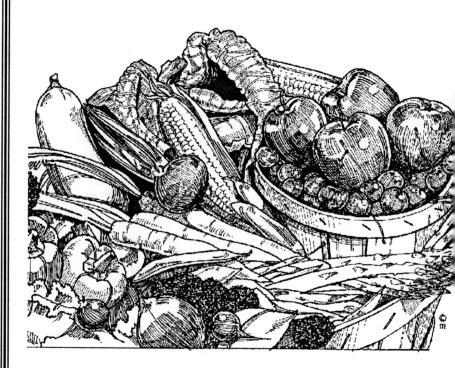

Chapter Six

Bowled Over by Beans

Protein packed and fiber rich, beans (legumes) can add a powerful wallop to your diet. As more and more people are looking towards a more vegetarian style diet, they are checking out the humble bean. Let me tell you about this under tooted legume. A legume is anything that comes in a pod that has an edible seed. This category includes soybeans and peanuts and all the more highly recognizable bean.

Legumes are an excellent source of complex carbohydrates, and are rich in the B vitamins, zinc, potassium, magnesium, calcium and iron. They are also more than 20 percent protein by dry weight. Because they are plants, they have no cholesterol, essentially no fat and very few calories. As a bonus, they are and excellent source of guar gum and pectin, two types of soluble fiber that have been shown to lower blood cholesterol.

Below are 20 different kinds of beans or legumes (there are more than 25 legumes available), all are great sources of nutrition.

Adzuki beans (also called azuki beans): Small, red and most commonly found in places that carry Asian foods. They are available as a red paste to which shortening and sugar have been added. Adzuki beans are often used in Asian desserts.

Black-eyed peas (also called cowpeas): These quick-cooking beans and their kissin' cousins, yellowed-eyed beans are small, oval, and creamy white, with either a black or a yellow spot. In the American South, they are the basis for the very popular hoppin' John, a "soul food" made with rice and typically served on New Year's Eve with the thought of bringing good luck for the new year.

Black beans (turtle beans): These beans are oval, about the size of a pea. A staple food in Latin America but also used extensively in many Asian dishes. They make wonderful soup, refried beans and sauces.

Cannellini: Large kidney-shaped white beans, often used in minestrone soup.

Chickpeas (garbanzos, ceci): Tan in color, about the size of a hazelnut. In fact, they have a nutty flavor. Popular in Middle Eastern dishes as well as Indian and Latin specialties, they form the basis of dishes such as humus, falafel and couscous.

Cranberry beans; Small beige ovals with pink spots; great in casseroles and soups.

Fava beans (broad beans): These look like big lima beans and are very popular in Italian dishes.

Flageolets: Pale green, baby kidney beans. French cooks love them.

Great Northern: The biggest of the white beans, they are kidney-shaped with a mild flavor.

Kidney beans: These beans come in many colors from red to white. They are great in chili, soups and on their own.

Lentils: Tiny beans available in many colors but come just one to a pod. Great in soups, the brown and green varieties are good in salads because they hold their shape after cooking.

Lima beans (Fordhooks, butter beans): These have had a difficult time with young eaters. Many of us probably spent our whole childhood avoiding them, but they now have come into their own as additions to soup, casseroles or mixed with other vegetables.

Mung beans: Usually found sprouted but are also available dried, mostly in health food and Asian markets. Because they are very small, they cook quite quickly.

Navy beans: The navy bean is small and whitish colored and is generally found in baked-bean recipes. Pork and beans, navy bean soup and Boston Baked Beans

Peanuts: A legume that grows in pods underground. Peanuts often are thought of as a nut. The oval, ivory-colored seeds are covered with a papery skin and encased in a fragile, tan pod. Peanuts have a buttery, nutty flavor when roasted.

Pinto bean: The most popular bean in the United States, and, in fact, they are the fiber champs of the legume family. When dried they look like they have been painted with red and tan specks.

Red beans: A favorite in the classic southern dish known as red beans and rice.

Soybeans: A staple food in Asia, often called the "cow of the East." Soybeans can be eaten fresh and dried. They are also used in making baby formula and their oil is used in salad dressings and margarine. Soy protein is widely used as a meat substitute and to enrich such foods as pasta and cereal. Soybeans have little flavor of their own so they can be used with other ingredients that have strong flavors.

Split peas: Great for soups because they cook quickly and have a distinctive taste. Split peas also make great purees and side dishes.

Whole Peas: These look like fresh garden peas that have been dried as is. They come in green and yellow, and can be used as a vegetable or as an ingredient in soups and casseroles.

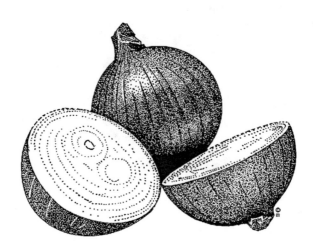

Chapter Seven

Seasonings by Herb

It has been a long time since I was first introduced to Herb or should I say herbs, like most people I was terrified that I would ruin my food by seasoning with herbs instead of just using salt and pepper. That of course is rarely true. Really if you look at the different types of seasonings and what they work well with you rarely go wrong. The key to teasing and tantalizing our palates with the flavors herbs imparts is to add them gently to begin with and add more to suit your own taste preferences. Herbs can improve bland recipes and change ordinary cuts of meat, vegetables or desserts into different and unusual dishes. Oregano for instance can replace salt, and tarragon when used with fish is known for removing most of the fishy taste. You will find that you will start using less salt in cooking when you rely on your friend herb.

A few tips on using herbs; fresh is best, but it is not always available. When using fresh herbs in a recipe you will need to use twice as much dried herbs, since the flavor of the fresh is less intense. Recently you have been able to buy some herbs in the freezer section, and those work much like the fresh herbs and can even be added frozen. Herbs should be kept in a cool, dry, dark cabinet away form the heat of your stove or refrigerator exhaust. Once a year, give dried herbs and ground spices the "sniff test" by passing the opened container quickly under your nose and seeing if the contents can be identified, if not discard the container and replace it. Whole spices will retain their flavor and aroma almost indefinitely.

To release the fullest flavor of fresh or dried herbs and seeds, crush them in the palm of your hand before adding them to the food. When only wanting to flavor long cooking dishes and not leave tell tell signs of herb being there try placing whole herbs in a old tea ball (that's my favorite tip) or tie them inside a piece of cheesecloth bag for easy removal. Since herbs do not hold well in lengthy cooking add them toward the end of cooking or if you added them at the beginning simply add an extra pinch to refresh the flavor just before the dish finishes cooking.

Now that I've given you a quick primer on how to use and store herbs here is a sample of various culinary herbs and spices with some suggestions for their uses. Use them in good health and taste.

Allspice: It has a delicate flavor that resembles a blend of cloves, cinnamon and nutmeg. Uses: pickles, meats, puddings, pies and drinks.

Anise: The flavor of anise is that of a sweet licorice taste: Uses: fruits, cakes, rolls, pie fillings, stews, and soups.

Basil: Has a mild, leafy, lemon flavor. Uses: tomato dishes, soups, also in squash and beans and sprinkled over meat.

Bay Leaves: Gives off a pungent, herbal flavor. Uses: vegetables, stews, seafoods, and soups.

Caraway: Has a flavor of rye bread. Uses: breads, cheese spreads, cookies, and vegetables, roast pork.

Cardamom: comes from the ginger family and has a bittersweet flavor. Uses: fruit, pastries, cakes, cookies, custards, sweet potatoes and pumpkin dishes.

Cayenne: Very Hot. Uses: Mexican cookery, chili, beef stews, cheese soufflés, and green vegetables.

Celery Seed: Tastes a lot like bitter celery. Uses: dips, soups, slaw, tomatoes, and salad dressings.

Chili Powder: Has a distinctive, hot spicy flavor. Uses: seafood, cocktails, soups, beans, Mexican cooking, and cheese sauces.

Chives: Have a mild green onion flavor. Uses: potatoes, sauces, dips and salads.

Cinnamon: Has a sweet, spicy flavor. Uses: cakes, cookies, puddings, fruit pies, spiced beverages and pumpkin dishes.

Cloves; Spicy, sweet, pungent flavor. Uses: ham, apples, pumpkin and mince pies, baked beans, teas, spice cake, cookies and puddings.

Coriander: From the parsley family, spicier. Uses: beans, salads, eggs, cheese, pork, sausage, curry sauce, rice and pickles.

Cumin: Salty, balsam like flavor. Uses: cheese spreads, deviled eggs, chicken, dressings, lamb, enchilada sauce, beans, breads and crackers.

Curry Powder: Exotic with heat. Uses: all Indian cooking, chicken, eggs, rice, vegetables and fish.

Dill: Similar to caraway, but milder and sweeter, has a slight bitter flavor. Uses: mostly in pickling, also in salads, soups, dips, fish, lamb, vegetables, eggs and cheeses.

Fenugreek: Has a maple flavor, not as sweet. Uses: Indian dishes, candies, cakes, cookies, and oriental cooking.

Garlic: From the onion family, it has a pungent flavor. Uses: dips, soups, vegetables, potatoes, meats, sauces, and bread.

Ginger: has a fragrant, hot, spicy sweet flavor. Uses: cookies, cakes, pies, puddings, applesauce, stews, fish, stuffing and oriental cooking.

Horseradish: Taste like parsnip, quite hot. Uses: dips, spreads, seafood, pork, lam, marinates, and cocktail sauces.

Mace: Similar to nutmeg. Uses: tomato juice, soups, fish, stews, pickling, gingerbread, cakes, welsh rarebit, chocolate dishes and fruit pies.

Marjoram: A delicate herbal flavor. Uses: soups, meats, eggs, sauces, and fish.

Mint: Has sweet leafy flavor. Uses: jelly, fruit salad, lam, and tea.

Mustard: A sharp, spicy flavor. Uses: salads, pickling, Chinese hot sauce, cheese sauce, vegetables, molasses cookies, fish and eggs.

Nutmeg: This has a sweet exotic flavor. Uses: doughnuts, eggnog, custards, spice cake, pumpkin, puddings, and sweet potatoes.

Oregano: A relative of marjoram, quite a bit stronger. Uses: pizza, spaghetti sauces, neat sauces, soups, vegetables and Italian specialties.

Paprika: A very mild taste, related to the bell pepper. Uses poultry, goulash, vegetables, soups, stews, salad dressings, meats and cream sauces.

Parsley: From the celery family, has a mild flavor. Uses: soups, salads, meat stews, all vegetables, and potatoes.

Pepper: Has a spicy, enduring aftertaste: Uses: most all foods except those with sweet flavors.

Peppermint: A strong minty flavor, quite soothing in tea. Uses: cream cheese spreads, coleslaw, lamb, garnishes, teas, and ices.

Poppy Seeds; A seed that is crunchy, and nutlike. Uses: breads, rolls, cookies, salads and cakes.

Rosemary: Has a delicate, sweetish taste. Uses: lamb dishes, coups, stews, beef, and fishes.

Saffron: Is a very strong, exotic spice, use sparingly. Uses; rice, breads, fish stew, chicken soup, cakes, fish sauces.

Sage: Has a strong flavor of camphoraceous and minty. Uses: meat and poultry, stuffing, sausages, meat loaf, hamburgers, stews and salads.

Savory: It has a mild pleasant taste. Uses: scrambled eggs, poultry, stuffing, hamburgers, fish, tossed salad, and tomatoes.

Sesame Seeds: has a crunchy, nutlike flavor. Uses: breads, rolls, cookies, candy, salad, fish, and asparagus.

Tarragon: This herb has a faint anise flavor. Uses: marinates for meats, poultry, omelets, fish, soups, and most vegetables.

Thyme: Has a strong, distinctive flavor. Uses: poultry seasoning, croquettes, fish, eggs, tomato dishes, and vegetables.

Turmeric: This comes from the ginger family and has a mild ginger-pepper flavor. Uses: pickles, salad dressings, rice and seafood.

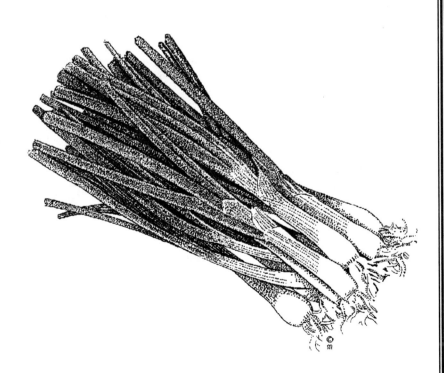

Seasonings by Herb

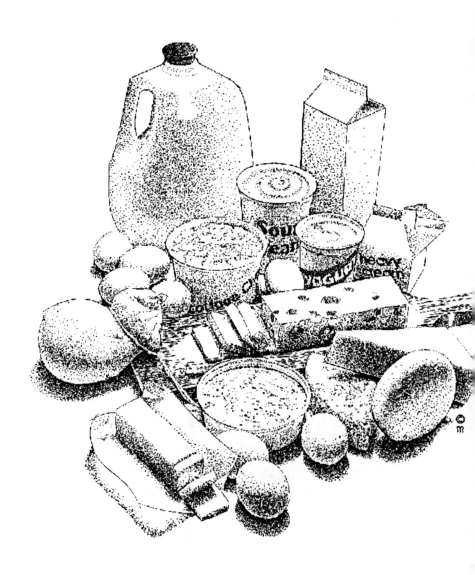

Chapter Eight

Mooove Over Dairy

D o you have a milk mustache?" My answer is NO! The fact is that milk has some pluses, but it is fattening, and it is a hidden element in many of our everyday foods. I once read that it takes as much energy for your body to digest eight ounces of whole milk as it does to digest eight ounces of steak. Wow! Did you also know that man is the only animal that drinks the milk of another species, and the only animal drinks milk after childhood, think about that.

Everybody has their own ideas about the importance of milk in our diets. When I began making changes in my diet the first thing to go was milk. That was very hard for a girl raised drinking fresh milk. I mean "fresh from the dairy milk," the kind you had to skim the cream off the top of the jar before you could use it. I actually felt like I was going through withdrawal symptoms when I just stopped drinking it, but I needed my body to put all of its attention into the healing process and not the pleasure of drinking a tall ice cold glass of milk everyday. One of the things I noticed that changed when I stopped drinking milk was no more gas. Yes, milk is one of those culprits that cause flatulence. Ice cream, oooh I just love ice cream and sometimes I just thought I would explode if I didn't get a big bowl of ice cream with all the fixings. It tasted so delightful until I was finished, then I would feel like I had a coating of fat stuck to the roof of my mouth. What a yucky feeling that was. Try and guess where all that fat is sticking inside of your body. I love ice cream, but like everyone else I also have to know my limitations. If I eat it everyday than all that fat sticks to my ribs (and thighs and stomach, etc.) and my energy level dive bombs.

Now not every type of milk product was off my list, I said good-bye to ice cream and glasses of milk, but not to cultured products like cheese and yogurt. It seems that the body reacts differently to fresh dairy products like milk, ice cream and butter than to cheese and yogurt because of the bacteria needed to create these items. Don't get the wrong idea, dairy products are not hideous monsters to be annihilated, but they do need to be kept in check, they are high in fats and calories.

Here are some items the Dairy Council produces in favor of milk products:

- *Dairy foods contain high-quality protein. Milk has all the essential amino acids, so it's as good as meat as a source of protein (my note - and as difficult to digest as meat).*
- *A small amount of milk protein, when combined with vegetable protein markedly boosts the nutritional quality of vegetable protein.*
- *Milk is a source of riboflavin, a B vitamin necessary to convert food into energy (my note - you can also get this great boost from certain vegetables). An eight-ounce glass of milk or a cup of yogurt provides 25 percent of your daily needs for this nutrient.*
- *Milk, yogurt and cheese are our body's best sources of calcium (my note - this is the dairy industry speaking. You can get as much calcium out of a serving of broccoli or spinach). Calcium helps build bone mass and maintain bone density and is an important mineral in preventing osteoporosis.*

- Milk is a nutrient-dense food. It contains significant amounts of nine nutrients, including protein, calcium, phosphorous, potassium, vitamin D, vitamin A, riboflavin, vitamin B 12 and carbohydrates.
- A cup of yogurt a day boost immune function and helps reduce the incidence and severity of colds, hay fever and other infections.

Here is some additional information about milk (not from the dairy council):

- Milk is a special food—the primary baby food, the first food of most mammals. It is considered our basic food of life, the connection between mother and child. Maybe that is why many of us develop a lifelong addiction to this sweet essence of life. Our love of sweet food, of which milk is our first, may be the reason why so many people accept and use sugar and sweet foods throughout their lives.
- Lactose, a simple sugar, should be easy to digest and use in our body for energy, but some children/adults may be unable to utilize this sugar; that is, they are lactose intolerant. Nearly half of the world population is lactose intolerant, which may cause bloating, abdominal pain, and diarrhea after milk is consumed.
- Milk is the most common food allergen. Milk allergies may manifest as skin rashes, eczema, chronic otitis media (fluid and/or infections in the ears), hyperactivity, and other problems.
- Homogenization is possibly the biggest concern in milk. It basically involves the blending of the milk fat into small globules so that it does not separate as it normally will do when it sits. It is possible that this process interferes with the body's ability to digest and utilize this fat in homogenized milk. The increase in cardiovascular disease has been correlated with the rise in the use of homogenized milk; however, further study is still needed to prove this relationship.

Are there alternatives to milk? Happily the answer is yes! I didn't really get introduced to the many other types of non-dairy beverages until we found out that my 10-month-old son was allergic to milk. At this point our doctor suggested we try a soy formula (formula having so many more added nutrients, than just straight soy beverage), but to our dismay we also found that the additional additives made my son's skin just as irritated as before. My friend JoAnne, brought over Rice, Soy, Multi-Grain and Oat beverages for us to try, then introduced us to a plethora of different types of non-dairy beverages. Each one had it's own horn to toot about which one would be the best nutritionally for him, but in the end my son decided he like the oat beverage. And boy how he likes it. If you want to get off the dairy-go-round you will find a large variety of beverages to try not just to put on your cereal in the morning but for cooking too.

Let's take a minute now to really look at the some of the different types of dairy and non-dairy products that are available. When we are finished I will give you some hints on how to cut the dairy fat out of your diets.

DAIRY PRODUCTS:

Acidophilus: Skim or low-fat milk that's made similarly to buttermilk, but with a different type of bacterial culture. Once the milk is drunk, the bacteria become active at body temperature, and doctors say that helps maintain the balance of beneficial microorganisms in the body's intestinal tract.

Butter: A dairy product made by churning cream skimmed from milk into a solid fat. In the United States, butter must be at least 80% milk fat.

Buttermilk: Milk, usually skim, to which special bacterial cultures are added. Buttermilk is smooth and fairly thick liquid, with a distinctive, slightly sour, tangy flavor. Dry buttermilk powder is also available.

Cheese: A dairy product made from heated milk with an enzyme or co-agulant added to form curds and whey. The curds are then pressed to form different shapes. Natural cheese is made directly from the curd and milk and not reprocessed or blended. Process cheese(to my way of thinking this is junk food, avoid it) is made from natural cheese, but it has undergone additional steps, such as pasteurization. Other ingredients are often added to enhance flavoring, a softer texture, and longer shelf life.

Cottage Cheese: Little Miss Muffet to like to eat a bowl of this (curds and whey), or a soft white, unripened, cow's milk cheese with a delicate but slightly acidic flavor. Early European farmers made this cheese in their "cottages" with the milk left over from making cheese. It is generally made from buttermilk or whey.

Cream Cheese: A white, fresh cheese with a smooth, dense and spreadable consistency, and a mild and slightly acidic flavor. This rich cheese is made from a mixture of cow's cream and milk. Available in several forms: regular, whipped, flavored, light and Neufchâtel.

Evaporated Milk: Whole milk from which 60 percent of the water has been removed. Evaporated low-fat (2%) and evaporated skim milk are also available.

Milk: Whole (3.5% fat or 150 calories per cup), 2% (2% fat or 120 calories per cup), 1% (1% fat or 102 calories per cup) and skim milk (0% fat or 86 calories per cup)

Nonfat Dry: Skim milk that has the water removed. This powdered form of milk reconstitutes easily in water. Nonfat dry milk is also known as powdered milk.

Sour Cream: A thick, smooth dairy product made by the action of a bacterial culture on cream. Most sour cream is made from sweet, light cream. There is also light and imitation sour creams available.

Sweetened Condensed Milk: Whole milk to which sugar is added and from which more than half the water is removed (make sure you see our lowfat/low sugar recipe on page 72).

Yogurt: A dairy product made by adding special bacterial cultures to milk (it can be whole milk, lowfat milk, or nonfat milk). Yogurt is thick and creamy with a tangy flavor.

NON-DAIRY PRODUCTS:

Almond Milk: A beverage made from grinding almonds and water together until it becomes smooth and creamy. It is then strained to create a very delicate tasting "milk".

Oat Milk: A smooth drink created by cooking water and oats together until smooth. It is then strained to make a heart healthy "milk". Low in fat, but sweet to the taste. Great in deserts. Available in original or vanilla.

    Rice Milk: A creamy liquid made by cooking 10 parts water to one part rice. After one hour it is pressed and strained to create "milk". Available in original, vanilla or chocolate.

    Soy Milk: A drink made from cooked soybeans that are especially useful for people with milk allergies. It comes in a variety of flavors like plain, vanilla and chocolate.

    Tofu: A cheeselike curd made from soybeans. Soybean curd or bean curd is made from soybean milk by a process similar to the one used for making cheese. Tofu is available in soft and firm style. The soft type is good for whipping, blending, and crumbling. Use firm tofu for slicing and cubing. A 1/2 cup serving contains about 95 calories, 10 grams of protein, 6 grams of fat and 0 cholesterol.

Tips and Hints for Cutting the Dairy Fat:

- *Switch to skim milk(or even a non-dairy milk). I know it reminds you of blue water, but the fat and calorie savings are significant. To make the switch begin gradually, downgrade from whole to 2 percent or 1 percent, if that is to difficult try combining the two, each time using a little more of the low-fat and a little less whole milk. Once you've made the switch to low fat milk, the whole milk will taste more like cream to you.*
- *Substitute evaporated skim milk for evaporated milk. When the recipe calls for cream use whole milk (unless it has to be whipped) or chilled evaporated skim milk (if whipping is necessary).*
- *In most recipes calling for sour cream, you can substitute plain low-fat yogurt and save yourself 349 calories per cup in the process. It is also a great substitute in salad dressings, dips and toppings for potatoes. Try replacing half the mayonnaise with yogurt. Soft tofu is also a great substitute in recipes calling for mayonnaise, sour cream or cream cheese, because it is tasteless and takes on the flavor of whatever seasonings you add to it.*
- *Blend low fat cottage cheese until smooth and use it to replace fat mayonnaise in your tuna salad, mixed with your favorite soup mix for dip or mixed into a sauce you need to be dairy smooth. It is also great put into a tossed green salad instead of fatty grated cheese or plopped onto a baked potato in place of sour cream.*

    I've presented a lot of information to you about dairy and non-dairy products alike, it is up to you to weigh it out and decide for yourself what will be best for you. The key here like everywhere else is *moderation*. If you want to continue to use dairy products, be smart about it and *use it in moderation*. A little can go a long way.

    In this book you will find I have offered you a choice of both dairy and non-dairy items alike. Because I have family members who are not only allergic to milk but are also lactose intolerant I generally lean more towards the non-dairy items, but only when taste, texture and the final product are not sacrificed.

Chapter Nine

Getting off the Fat-Go-Round

To eat fat or not to eat fat that —is the question. Whether 'tis nobler to suffer the bulging thighs and waistline caused by consuming too much fat or to fight the good fight of reducing my intake I do not know (My apologies to Mr. Shakespeare). You get the point though. I think that dealing with fat is the number one cry of people striving to lead healthier lives. How do I get the fat out!

First off, we need to stop looking at fat as the latest health food craze or fad. I remember not to many years ago when the idea was to make everything fat free, then it changed to minimum fats and now it is just to lower fat intake. With all these changes over the past several years, it is no wonder our society is confused and getting fatter on all the reduced fat stuff out there. If you pick up a package of reduced fat cookies and look at the labeling there is either a small amount of fat or no fat. Okay, so the fat is gone but what did they replace it with? Are you ready for this ... sugar. That's right, your fat is being replaced by sugar, therefore you may be eating less fat but you are eating more carbohydrates (more calories) in every bite. But since there is no fat we think we can eat more and when we do we consume more calories. No wonder we are on a fat-go-round and as America tries to cut the fats in our diets we are getting fatter. What is that old saying, "Stop the boat! I want to get off!"

There are three types of fats - the good, the bad and the ugly or another way to put that is monounsaturated, polyunsaturated and saturated. You need to know the difference between fats.

First, the "good" fat, called monounsaturated, comes from vegetable sources and includes olive and canola oils. Diets high in monounsaturated have been found to reduce blood cholesterol levels as much as a low-fat diet does and also improve the ratio of HDL (good) cholesterol to LDL (bad) which can cut the risk of hardening of the arteries. That doesn't mean that you can pour on the oil, moderation is still the best bet

Second, some foodstuffs contain a "bad" fat, called polyunsaturated. It comes also from vegetable sources, which include safflower, sunflower, corn, sesame, soybean and peanut oils. Polyunsaturates were always thought be the best kind of fat because they lower cholesterol. But recent studies indicate that certain types of polyunsaturates raise fat levels. Watch out for hydrogenated or partially hydrogenated polyunsaturated fats. The process of hydrogenization is used to convert oils to solid form or to better the texture of processed foods or increase their shelf life.

Third, the "ugly" fat called saturated fat is easily recognizable because it is solid at room temperature. These include such culprits as palm kernel oil, coconut oil and animal fats such as meat, eggs, dairy, butter and lard which have been shown to raise serum cholesterol levels. To give you a clue about the negative nature of solid fats; in the early 1940's, the government-needed materials for bombs, and one such ingredient, glycerin, was in short supply. Fats (used greases and cooking oils) were a source of glycerin, so ingenuity took over. People proudly saved their household grease and cooking oils so that they could dump the strained grease into large barrels. These barrels were then take to manufacturing plants where the glycerin was extracted and used to make "headaches for Hitler." I guess you could say they were "fat conscious."

Fats, like carbohydrates, are composed of carbon, hydrogen, and oxygen. They are the most concentrated source of food energy supplying nine calories per gram. Fat transports the fat-soluble vitamins A, D, E, and K and is the source of the essential fatty acids necessary for normal growth. Whether we like it or not we do need a certain amount of good fat in our diets because it is necessary for the production of a variety of body compounds including hormone-like substances called prostaglandin which control a vast range of bodily functions.

The typical American diet contains 42% of calories from fat. Just imagine your 42% of your plate piled up with that yellowy chicken fat. Isn't that disgusting … yuck! The American Heart Association and the American Cancer Society recommend no more than 30% of calories be derived from fat, and saturated fat intake should be less than 10% of calories. Excessive fat consumption is a primary risk factor for heart disease and stroke, cancer and obesity. In *For Health's Sake* I have tried to make sure that all the recipes are low in saturated fat and contain 30% or less (mostly less) of it's calories from fat.

What is the key to fat control? Moderation, not fads. If you want fat free foods learn how to use substitutions (see page 47) that increase taste and not fat content. Don't let fat control you … you control fat. Dr. Robert Haaas once stated, "Why eat large amounts of the very substance - fat - you are trying to burn?"… It is about time you learned the truth: to lose weight, spare muscle, and achieve blood chemistry values in the peak performance range *concentrate on complex carbohydrates*. Our prehistoric ancestors thrived on them - and so will you!" That goes back to what I have said in previous chapters. Eat your fruits, vegetables and grains and put meats, eggs, dairy and fats on the back burner. This is something you can do and will do for more energy and better health.

I like what Mark Twain had to say, "Some habits must be eased downstairs a step at a time." How you do that easing and to what degree is up to you. That is why I listed some of my favorite books on fat reduction in the section *My Favorite Books* on page 201. In the meantime just look at the following easy ideas for controlling the fat in your diet:

- *Build your meals around vegetables and grains and use meat as the condiment. This will not only keep your fat in check, but will help you avoid over consuming protein.*
- *Replace the oil called for in baked goods with thick purees such as applesauce, pears, apricots or prunes.*
- *Replace oil for sautéing with broth or juice. Better yet have a variety of different flavored vegetable cooking sprays.*
- *Use good Teflon baking pans — they will help reduce the amount of oil needed in cooking.*
- *Replace shortening or oils in baking with an equal volume of pureed fruit and 1/3 of the oil called for.*
- *Replace some of the whole eggs called for with two egg whites. Each egg replaced with two egg whites will save five grams of fat. It's usually a good*

idea to keep at least one or two whole eggs to maintain the correct taste and consistency. For example, replace 3 whole eggs with 1 whole egg and 4 egg whites —you'll save 10 grams of fat. Try egg substitutes like flax seed eggs (found on page 58) Just Whites or Egg Beaters.

- *Use low fat milk and cheese products or better still switch to non-dairy substitutes like soy, oat, almond or rice milk.*
- *Eat fat free yogurt and use it instead of sour cream in baking dips and sauces.*
- *Develop a fear of frying.*
- *Toast nuts. This intensifies the flavor so you don't have to use as many.*
- *When you must use fats, use polyunsaturated vegetable oils. My favorites are canola, safflower and corn. Corn oil also gives foods a buttery taste without the butter.*

I hope you will take these tips to heart and apply them into your lives. Remember - Fat ain't where it's at! Making the decision to change to a healthy lifestyle is hard sometimes. Don't forget to congratulate yourself from time to time on your progress, take time to smell the roses and enjoy how much better you feel now.

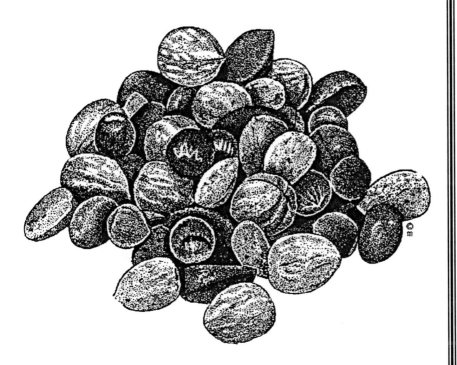

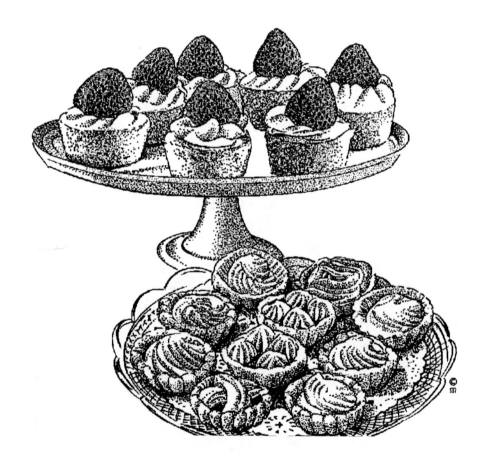

Chapter Ten

The Truth about Sweeteners

Sugar, sweeteners, honey ... call it what you will; if it is sweet we need to use it in *moderation*. Most of us have very little knowledge of all the different kinds of sweeteners in the world today. Natural, artificial and refined sweeteners can improve the flavor and pleasure of many of the foods we eat. If you look at a food label you will undoubtedly see the words glucose, dextrose, maltose, sucrose, aspartame along with a number of other words used for sugar. You might be surprised to see amount of sugar listed say in peanut butter or the ever-popular Snack Wells™ cookies or even in spaghetti sauce. We have become a nation of sugar addicts, more apt to grab a sugar-laden treat than a piece of tasty fruit. Regardless of what kind of sweetener you use, sugar is sugar and your body absorbs it just like any other type of carbohydrate you eat. All carbohydrates are converted to a sugar in the intestines, so if you eat a potato or a candy bar you body will treat it the same. "The rise in blood sugar after meals depends on total carbohydrates eaten, not on the types".

The following is a list of some of the most common sweeteners and their attributes, you may be surprised at what you read, but here is the truth about sweeteners.

Aspartame - is also known as NutraSweet™ and Equal™; a chemical combination of the two amino acids aspartic acid and phenylalanie. Although made from two natural ingredients, aspartame is not found in nature.

Barley Malt - a mild sweetener produced by sprouting the grain, which forms sugars (maltose), contains trace amounts of nutrients; available as granules or syrup.

Brown Rice Syrup - a mild sweetener produced similar to barley malt.

Brown Sugar - a processed mixture of granulated sugar and molasses that is moist when fresh. Light brown sugar has less molasses flavor and dark brown sugar has more.

Confectioners' Sugar - is also known as powdered sugar. This is refined white granulated sugar that has been pulverized. Manufactures usually add a small amount of cornstarch to prevent caking.

Date Sugar - dried, pulverized dates; a whole food sweetener rich in beta carotene, B 1, magnesium and phosphorus; does not dissolve well but good for sprinkling on cereal, fruit, baked goods.

Fructose - a refined sugar; one component of sucrose and one third sweeter; also called levulose or fruit sugar. Fructose is metabolized more slowly than sucrose and does not drive up the blood sugar as quickly. A true fructose comes in a crystalline form. It is generally corn derived but <u>not</u> from corn syrup. Make sure you buy crystalline type fructose otherwise you are just buying sugar.

Fruit Juice Concentrate - made by evaporating fruit juice; apple, orange and pineapple are found in the frozen food section of your grocery stores.

Glucose - also called dextrose, corn sugar or grape sugar; one component of sugar, raises the blood sugar more quickly than any other sugar.

Glycerin - a syrupy liquid derived from fats; 60% as sweet as sugar. Glycerin is converted directly into glycogen (store sugar) thus it does not usually trigger a pancreatic reaction as does sugar. Some individuals may be allergic to glycerin.

Honey - a natural sweetener with trace amounts of nutrients. The darker the color, the stronger the flavor

Lactose - milk sugar, not as sweet as sucrose or glucose; about 20% of the U.S. Population is lactose intolerant.

Maple Syrup/Sugar - made from the sap of maple trees; high in minerals; syrup is graded according to color and strength of flavor. Maple flavored syrups may contain as little as 3% maple syrups, the rest being corn syrup (glucose and fructose).

Molasses - is a by product of the sugar refining process and an ingredient in gingerbread. Molasses has a strong flavor and is a rich food source for iron and other minerals.

Sorghum - a plant related to the millet family; stalks are crushed to render a sweet juice, which is boiled down. Sorghum syrup is similar to, but milder in flavor than maple syrup.

Stevia - a liquid herbal sweetener also known as honeyleaf, thirty to forty times sweeter than sugar. Stevia does not promote tooth decay and may even prove effective for the prevention of cavities. Is only available in a whole food or health food store.

Sucant - stands for "sugar cane natural", the dehydrated juice of organically grown sugar cane in granular form; contains up to 3% mineral salts, vitamins and trace mineral (brown and turbinado sugars contain only 0.5% mineral salts) My favorite brand is Florida Crystals and it comes in three varieties: Milled Cane, Demerara & Muscovado.

Sucrose - White refined table sugar; cheapest most commonly used sweetener. Like all refined sugars, sucrose lacks the nutrients (vitamins, minerals, and fiber) required to metabolize it properly in the body. The average American consumes 150 pounds a year.

Turbinado Sugar - also known as raw sugar, another form of sucant.

Xylitol, Inositol, Mannitol, Sorbitol - four closely related natural sugar substitutes (occurring in plants) that do not cause insulin release. Excessive amounts can cause diarrhea.

We need to eliminate or at the very least greatly reduce concentrated carbohydrates which contain excessive amounts of sugar that can overload our bloodstream with glucose, like candy, cookies and cakes, etc.. These sweets contain not only the white sugar that takes the B vitamins from our systems but also artificial preservatives that make the liver toxic and irritate the mucus lining of the intestines.

What does this all boil down to? Make it yourself whenever possible so you can control the type and amount of sweetener you use. Most recipes can have their sugar content reduced by 1/4 to 1/3 and still be plenty sweet. You will find that as you cut back on your sweeteners that the next time you have a cookie from the bakery that it will actually taste too sweet to you.

Rule of thumb - IF IT TASTES SWEET USE MODERATION. That is the key to good eating ... *moderation.*

Chapter Eleven

Oh No I'm Out of ...
A Guide to Substitutions

J ust imagine that you are in the middle of making your world famous dessert and you've got guests arriving in one hour. You open the cupboards to get your favorite seasoning and discover much to your chagrin that you are all out, argh, now what do you do? At one time or another we have all been in this situation and cannot stop what we are doing to run to the store to get the proper ingredient. What do you do? Do you panic, no, you turn to your handy dandy substitution list, most cookbooks have one, and you fix your problem.

Do you get a substandard product by making substitutions?

Not hardly.

In fact, it's likely you won't notice a difference in the presentation or from anybody who is consuming your culinary fare. Truthfully, unless you tell them they won't even know that there is a difference. Substitutions go to new heights today with the advent of low fat and low sugar cooking. Hopefully I can give you the best of both worlds in the lists below.

Spices and Herbs

Allspice, ground (1 teaspoon): 1/2 teaspoon cinnamon and 1/4 teaspoon each nutmeg and ground cloves.

Capers: Chopped green olives.

Cayenne Pepper (1/8 teaspoon): 4 drops hot pepper sauce.

Chives, fresh: Green onions, including the tops.

Cilantro: Fresh Italian parsley (for looks only) or parsley with a touch of lemon juice, to taste.

Cumin (t teaspoon): 1/3 teaspoon ground anise plus 2/3 teaspoon ground caraway seeds.

Fine herbs: Equal parts chervil, chives, tarragon and parsley.

Five-spice powder: Equal parts cinnamon, cloves, fennel seed, star anise and Szechwan peppercorns.

Fresh herbs minced (1 tablespoon): 1 teaspoon dried, of the same kind.

Ginger, candied (1 tablespoon): 1/8 teaspoon ground ginger.

Ginger, dried (1 teaspoon): 1/4 teaspoon ground ginger.

Garlic, fresh (1 small clove): 1/8 teaspoon garlic powder; 1/4 teaspoon minced dried.

Horseradish, fresh grated (1 tablespoon): 2 tablespoons prepared, well drained.

Italian seasoning: Oregano, marjoram, thyme, basil, rosemary and sage.

Lemon grass, minced (1 tablespoon): 1 teaspoon grated lemon rind.

Mustard, dried (1 teaspoon): 1 tablespoon prepared mustard.

Pumpkin pie spice (1 teaspoon): 1/2 teaspoon cinnamon mixed with 1/8 teaspoon each: ground ginger, nutmeg, mace and cloves.

Saffron (1/8 teaspoon): 1/2 to 1 teaspoon turmeric (for color only).

Shallots: Minced onion with half a small clove of minced garlic.

Szechwan peppercorns: Five-spice powder.

Vanilla bean: 1 teaspoon vanilla extract.

Baking Ingredients

Arrowroot (1 1/2 teaspoons): 1 tablespoon flour or cornstarch.

Baking powder (1 teaspoon): 1/4 teaspoon baking soda and 5/8 teaspoon cream of tartar.

Chocolate, semi-sweet (1 ounce): 1/2 ounce unsweetened chocolate plus 1 tablespoon sugar.

Chocolate, unsweetened (1 ounce): 3 tablespoons cocoa powder plus 1 tablespoon butter.

Cornstarch (1 tablespoon): 2 tablespoons all-purpose flour or 1 tablespoon arrowroot.

Corn syrup (1 cup): 1 1/4 cups sugar plus 1/3 cup water. Boil until syrupy.

Currants, dried: Chopped dark raisins.

Eggs (1 whole): 2 egg whites; 4 teaspoons powdered egg whites, 1 teaspoon cornstarch and 3 tablespoons water, 2 tablespoons tofu, 1 tablespoon flax seed eggs (see recipe on page 58) or 1 tablespoon gelatin eggs (see recipe on page 74).

Flour, all-purpose (1 cup): 1 cup plus 2 tablespoons cake flour.

Flour, sifted cake (1 cup): 3/4 cup plus 2 tablespoons sifted all-purpose flour.

Flour, self-rising (1 cup): 1 cup all-purpose flour plus 1 1/2 teaspoons baking powder and 1/8 teaspoon salt.

Flour, whole-wheat (1 cup): 2 tablespoons wheat germ plus enough white flour to make 1 cup.

Fructose: 1 tablespoon of granulated sugar is equal to 2 teaspoons of fructose, 1/2 cup granulated sugar is equal to 5 tablespoons of fructose, 1 cup granulated sugar is equal to 2/3 cup fructose. This is the standard substitution although I find that 3/4 cup is a more suitable substitution. You can find fructose in the sugar or diabetic section of your grocery store or at your local health or whole foods store.

Graham cracker crumbs (1 cup): 15 graham crackers, ground in a food process or 1 cup vanilla wafer crumbs.

Honey (1 cup): 1 1/4 cups sugar plus 1/4 cup more liquid than required in recipe (this may cause product to brown faster and necessitate a lower oven temperature).

Lemon juice (1 teaspoon): 1/2 teaspoon vinegar.

Marshmallow cream (7 ounces): 1 (16 ounce) package marshmallows, melted, plus 3 1/2 tablespoons light corn syrup.

Molasses: 3/4 cup brown sugar plus 1/4 cup water.

Orange peel, dried (1 tablespoon): 1 1/2 teaspoon orange extract: 1 tablespoon grated orange zest.

Orange peel, grated: Orange marmalade, or lemon or lime peel.

Pecans, chopped (1 cup): 1 cup regular oats, toasted in 350° oven until golden.

Pine nuts: Walnuts or almonds

Shortening: When substituting vegetable oil for vegetable shortening, butter or margarine, use one-third less. Use 2 teaspoons of oil in place of 1 tablespoon of hard shortening.

Sugar, confections (1 cup): 1 cup sugar plus 1 tablespoon cornstarch processed in a food processor fitted with the metal blade.

Sugar, light brown (1 cup): 1/2 cup each dark brown sugar and white sugar or 1/4 cup light molasses and 1 cup white sugar.

Sugar, superfine: Granulated sugar processed until powder.

Sugar, white granulated (1 cup): 1 cup firm-packed brown sugar; 2 cups confections sugar, sifted; 3/4 cup honey (reduce liquid by 1/4 cup or add 1/4 cup flour); 1 1/4 cups molasses (reduce liquid in recipe by 1/4 cup or add 1/4 cup additional flour if no other liquid is called for); 1 cup frozen fruit juice concentrate (reduce liquid by same amount); 1 1/4 cup barley malt syrup (use a 1/4 cup less liquid) or 1/2 cup brown rice syrup.

Tamarind paste (1 tablespoon): 1 teaspoon each minced dates, prunes and dried apricots plus 1 teaspoon lemon juice.

Tapioca (1 tablespoon): 1 1/2 tablespoons flour.

Yeast, cake (5/8 ounce): 1 packet active dry yeast.

Yeast (1 package): 1 tablespoon dry yeast.

Dairy Products
Butter (1 cup): 1 cup margarine, 7/8 cup vegetable shortening; 7/8 cup corn oil; 1 cup shortening, or 1 cup applesauce for baking or 1 cup orange or apple juice concentrate for baking.

Buttermilk (1 cup): 1 tablespoon vinegar or lemon juice plus enough milk to equal 1 cup, allowed to stand 5 minutes; 1 cup milk plus 1 3/4 tablespoons cream of tartar plus 1 1/2 teaspoons lemon juice, allowed to stand 5 minutes or 1 cup plain low-fat yogurt.

Cheddar cheese: American, Colby, longhorn or soy cheddar cheese.

Cream cheese: Blend 1 cup low-fat cottage cheese with 1/4 cup margarine to each 1 cup cream cheese that is lower in saturated fat and cholesterol (but not lower in total fat); 1 cup soft tofu.

Crème fraiche (1 cup): 1 cup whipping cream with 2 tablespoons buttermilk, mixed in a glass container and allowed to stand at room temperature until thick, 8-24 hours. Stir; refrigerate up to 10 days.

Evaporated Milk (1 cup): 1 cup water and 2/3 cup instant nonfat dry milk or powdered soy milk.

Half-and-half: 7/8 cup whole milk plus 1 1/2 tablespoons butter.

Farmer's cheese: Dry curd cottage cheese.

Sour cream (1 cup): 1 cup plain yogurt; 1 cup buttermilk; 1 cup evaporated milk plus 1 tablespoon vinegar; 1 cup cottage cheese pureed with 2 tablespoons milk and 1 tablespoon lemon juice or whip 1/2 cup of *chilled* evaporated milk with 1 tablespoon of white vinegar to equal 1 cup.

Whole milk (1cup): 1/2 cup evaporated milk plus 1/2 cup water; 1 cup reconstituted nonfat dry milk plus 2 teaspoons oil; 1 cup skim milk plus 2 teaspoons oil; 1 cup soymilk plus 2 teaspoons melted butter. In most recipes for cakes and muffins, fruit juice can be used in place of milk (and sugar, see sugar substitutes above). Add 1/2 teaspoon of baking soda to the recipe if the juice is acidic.

Yogurt (cup): 1 cup buttermilk.

Miscellaneous
Bacon: In place of this high-fat ingredient, use lean Canadian bacon or boiled or baked ham or soy bacon.

Beef broth (1 cup): 1 bouillon cube plus one cup of water or 1 teaspoon beef soup base plus one cup boiling water.

Bread crumbs (1 cup): 3/4 cup of cracker or cereal crumbs; 1 cup wheat germ or 1 cup oatmeal.

Chicken broth (1 cup): 1 bouillon cube plus one cup of water or 1 teaspoon chicken soup base plus one cup boiling water.

Chili sauce: Ketchup with prepared horseradish and lemon juice.

Hot sauce: Crushed red pepper flakes.

Ketchup (3/4 cup): 3/4 cup chili sauce or 1/2 cup tomato sauce plus 3 tablespoons sugar and tablespoon white vinegar.

Prepared mustard (1 tablespoon): 1 teaspoon dry mustard mixed with 2 teaspoons wine vinegar, white wine or water.

Tahini (sesame paste): Smooth peanut butter plus sesame seed oil to taste.

Tomato juice (1 cup): 2 or 3 fresh ripe tomatoes, peeled, seeded and pureed with salt and lemon juice to taste; 1/2 cup tomato sauce plus 1/2 cup water.

Tomato sauce (1 cup): 3/8 cup tomato paste and 1/2 cup water.

Vinegar (1/2 teaspoon): 1 teaspoon lemon juice.

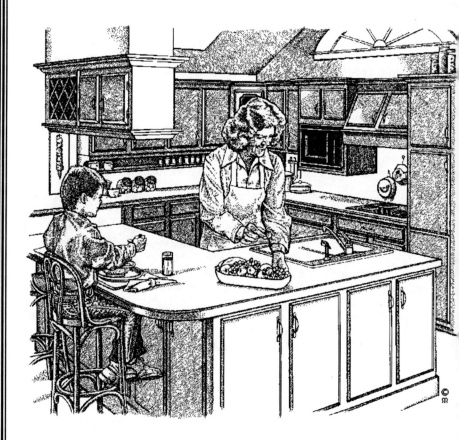

Appetizers, Beverages and So Forth

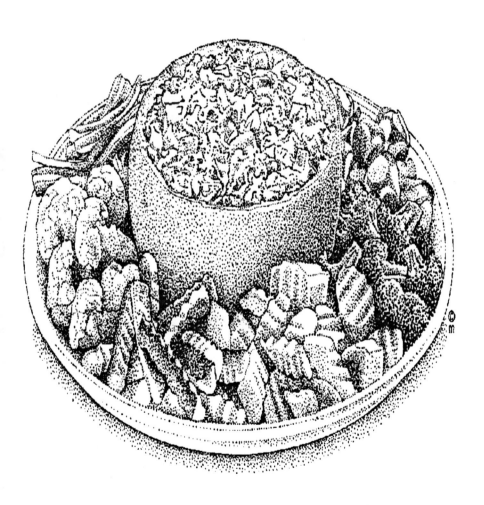

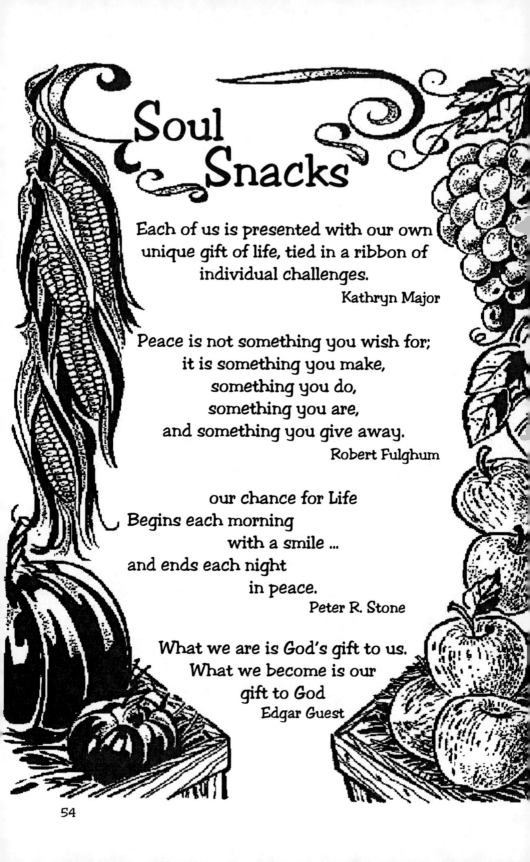

Soul Snacks

Each of us is presented with our own
unique gift of life, tied in a ribbon of
individual challenges.

Kathryn Major

Peace is not something you wish for;
it is something you make,
something you do,
something you are,
and something you give away.

Robert Fulghum

our chance for Life
Begins each morning
with a smile ...
and ends each night
in peace.

Peter R. Stone

What we are is God's gift to us.
What we become is our
gift to God

Edgar Guest

Seven Layer Bean Dip

*When I make this there is never enough. Plan on this dish disappearing fast.
Some times this becomes a main dish in our house, served with steaming
corn on the cob.*

1	**cup fat-free refried beans**
1 1/2	**cups guacamole (optional)**
1	**cup sour cream, light**
1 1/2	**cups salsa**
4	**ounces black olives, drained and sliced**
1	**cup green onion, chopped**
1	**cup shredded lowfat cheddar cheese**
	Baked tortilla chips

In a large flat serving dish with at least 2-inch sides (like a glass quiche pan)
spread beans. Then place a layer of guacamole, followed by a layer of sour
cream and salsa. Sprinkle black olives and green onions over sour cream and
top with shredded cheddar or co-jack cheese. Serve with tortilla chips.

Variation on a Theme
You can save on your fat calories by eliminating the guacamole. In it's place
try adding a layer of sliced Galapagos or shredded lettuce and diced tomatoes.
This is a great dish anytime.

Yield:: 20

🍎🍎🍎🍎🍎

Per serving: 52 Calories; 3g Fat (satfat 0.7g); 3g Protein; 5g Carbohydrate;
2mg Cholesterol; 207mg Sodium

Baked Tortilla Chips

12	**corn tortillas, extra thin**
	vegetable oil spray

Heat oven to 400°F. Cut tortillas into quarters. Spray on both sides with cooking spray. Place in single layer on 1 or 2 baking sheets. Bake until edges turn
crisp and golden, about 10 to 12 minutes.

Yield 4-6 servings.

Variation on a Theme
Try different flavored vegetable oil sprays, or try sprinkling chili powder or garlic

powder on chips before baking them. Be bold. Also works on flour tortillas.

🍎🍎🍎🍎🍎

Per serving: 166 Calories; 2g Fat (satfat 0.2g); 4g Protein; 35g Carbohydrate;
0mg Cholesterol; 121mg Sodium

Calcutta

8	whole prunes
1	tablespoon chutney
3	tablespoons brown rice, cooked
1	minced gherkins
1/8	teaspoon salt
1/8	teaspoon paprika
	Worcestershire sauce
8	slices turkey bacon

Select large prunes; cook till tender; remove seeds. Mix together chutney, rice, gherkin, salt and paprika. Stuff rice mixture into prunes, then dip in Worcester-shire sauce; wrap each stuffed prune with a slice of turkey bacon; fasten with toothpick. Broil until bacon is crisp. Serve hot.
Yield::   8 servings

🍎🍎🍎🍎🍎

Per serving: 63 Calories; 1g Fat (satfat 0.1; 5g); Protein; 10g Carbohydrate; 9mg Cholesterol; 357mg Sodium

Chi Tan Chuan (Chinese Egg Rolls)

1	package won-ton wrappers
1	egg, beaten
1/3	cup celery, finely diced
1/4	cup water chestnuts, minced
1/4	cup bamboo shoots, chopped
1/4	cup bean sprouts
1	tablespoon tamari soy sauce
1	cup sausage, browned and drained
	or chopped shrimp, lobster, or crab meat
	oil for frying

Brown sausage, rinse and drain. Mix 1 egg and remaining ingredients. Place 1 heaping tablespoon into center of won-ton wrapper. Fold wrapper in on either side then roll up, tucking in edges to seal in fillings. A little water can be used for sealing. Chill. Just before serving brown in 2" of hot fat. You can spray these with vegetable spray and bake in the oven at 425° F for 5 minutes or until browned. A suggestion for serving might be setting a bowl of Chinese Sauce or Sweet and Sour Sauce in a bowl for dipping egg rolls in.
Yield: 30 egg rolls

🍎🍎🍎🍎🍎

Per serving: 37 Calories; 3g Fat (satfat 1.2g); 1g Protein; 1g Carbohydrate; 11mg Cholesterol; 84mg Sodium

Celery Pinwheels

| 1 | bunch celery |
| 1 | cup Nicole's Favorite Herb and Garlic Cheese (page 57) |

Separate stalks from 1 bunch of celery. Fill each stalk with Nicole's Favorite Herb and Garlic Cheese. Put stalks back together; tie firmly together with rubber bands and chill.   Slice crosswise 1/4 to 1/2 inch thick.
Yield 24 - 36 pinwheels.

🍎🍎🍎🍎🍎

Per serving: 0 Calories; less than one gram Fat (satfat 0.1g); 0g Protein; 0g Carbohydrate; 0mg Cholesterol; 1mg Sodium

Devilish Eggs

If you're craving deviled eggs try these lower fat ones. The total fat is still high as long is there are yolks in eggs, but these are considerably lower in fat than the old way.

2	large eggs, hard-boiled
1/4	cup lowfat cottage cheese *or* silken tofu
1	tablespoon plain nonfat yogurt *or* soy yogurt
1/4	teaspoon mustard powder
	pinch turmeric
	fresh ground pepper to taste
	paprika

Shell eggs, cut in half lengthwise, and remove the yolks. In a small bowl, combine cottage cheese, yogurt, mustard, turmeric and pepper. Blend until smooth with a small wire whisk. Spoon mixture into cavities of eggs. Sprinkle very lightly with paprika. *Yield:* 4

🍎🍎🍎🍎🍎

Per serving: 44 Calories; 2g Fat (48% calories from fat); satfat 0.8; 5g Protein; 1g Carbohydrate; 91mg Cholesterol; 87mg Sodium

Guacamole
Serve as a dip with chips or crackers.

3	whole avocados
1	tablespoon onion minced
2	whole jalepeno peppers, canned, seeded
1	whole fresh tomatoes chopped
1	tablespoon fresh coriander leaf, chopped
1/2	teaspoon salt
1	pinch black pepper
1	tablespoon fresh lemon juice
1	dash Tabasco sauce
1	tablespoon sour cream, light

Peel avocados, cut them in halves and remove pits. Toss with lemon juice in a ceramic bowl. Mash with a fork until smooth. Add remaining ingredients, blend well, and adjust seasoning to taste.

Yield: 8 servings (1 serving equals 2 tablespoons)

🍎🍎🍎🍎🍎

Per serving: 102 Calories; 9g Fat (satfat 1.4g); 2g Protein; 7g Carbohydrate; 0mg Cholesterol; 643mg Sodium

Nicole's Favorite Herb and Garlic Cheese

I first tried herb and garlic style cheeses when I visited France and loved them. I soon discovered Alouette and a few other European styles of this cheese but they were expensive. So I tried making my own and my daughter loves it so much, she called it her favorite cheese. I think you will like it too!

8	ounces fat-free cream cheese or silken tofu
1	tablespoon herb and garlic salad dressing mix
2	tablespoons milk, skim or soy milk

In a food processor with a steel blade place cream cheese and 1 tablespoon of herb and garlic salad dressing mix and 1 tablespoon milk. Blend until smooth. Check for consistency. Cheese should be spreadable. If it is still to thick add another tablespoon of milk.

Yield: 8 (Yield: is 2 tablespoons)

Variation on a Theme

Try other flavors of seasoning with cream cheese, like Italian. The combinations are endless.

🍎🍎🍎🍎🍎

Per serving: 31 Calories; 0g Fat (satfat 0g); 4g Protein; 2g Carbohydrate; 4mg Cholesterol; 157mg Sodium

Salmon Log

1	can salmon, canned
8	ounces fat-free cream cheese
1	tablespoon lemon juice
2	tablespoons onion grated
1	teaspoon horseradish mustard
1/4	teaspoon salt
1	teaspoon liquid Barbecue Smoke®
1/3	cup walnuts, finely chopped
3	tablespoons parsley, chopped

Drain and flake salmon, removing skin and bones. Combine salmon with cream cheese, lemon juice, onion, horseradish, salt and liquid smoke; mix well. Chill several hours. Combine walnuts and parsley. Shape salmon mixture into an 8x2-inch log. Roll log in nut mixture. Chill well. Serve with crisp crackers as an hors d'oeurve.

Yield: about 16 1/2-inch slices.

Variation on a Theme

Try using the same amount of tuna in place of the salmon. To lose a few more fat grams and calories skip the walnuts and roll in a mixture of parsley and toasted sesame seeds.

🍎🍎🍎🍎🍎🍎

Per serving: 34 Calories; 1g Fat (satfat 0.5g); 4g Protein; 1g Carbohydrate; 7mg Cholesterol; 173mg Sodium

Stuffed Cucumbers

2	large cucumber
1	cup tuna in water
2	tablespoons light mayonnaise or tofu
1/2	teaspoon onion, grated
1/2	teaspoon lemon juice
1/2	teaspoon Worcestershire sauce
	salt and pepper to taste

Remove center of cucumbers with apple corer, set aside. Mix together tuna, mayonnaise, onion, lemon juice, Worcestershire sauce, salt and pepper. Stuff mixture into center of cucumber; place in refrigerator to chill. Just before serving cut crosswise into 1/2-inch slices.

Yield: 36 1/2-inch slices.

🍎🍎🍎🍎🍎🍎

Per serving: 9 Calories; less than one gram Fat (satfat 0g); 1g Protein; 1g Carbohydrate; 2mg Cholesterol; 22mg Sodium

Vegetable Dip

1	tablespoon chives, freeze-dried
1/2	teaspoon dill weed
1	teaspoon garlic salt
1/2	teaspoon paprika
1	teaspoon lemon juice
1	cup tofu or light sour cream

Combine all ingredients in a small bowl until evenly distributed.
Yield: 16 (Yield: is equal to 2 tablespoons)

🍎🍎🍎🍎🍎

Per serving: 10 Calories; 1g Fat (satfat 0.2g); 1g Protein; 0g Carbohydrate;

0mg Cholesterol; 2mg Sodium

Cherry/Apple Drink

2	envelopes powdered drink mix, cherry
1/2	cup fructose
6	ounces lemonade, frozen concentrate thawed
1 1/2	quarts ice water

Combine ingredients; stir until fructose is dissolved.
Yield: 24 servings

🍎🍎🍎🍎🍎

Per serving: 25 Calories; 0g Fat (satfat 0g); 0g Protein; 7g Carbohydrate; 0mg
Cholesterol; 2mg Sodium

Citrus Refresher

2	6 ounce lemonade, frozen concentrate, thawed
1	6 ounce orange juice, frozen concentrate, thawed
2	cups pineapple juice
3 1/2	quarts ice water

Combine ingredients in order given.
Yield: 27 servings

🍎🍎🍎🍎🍎

Per serving: 52 Calories; less than one gram Fat (satfat 0g); 0g Protein; 13g
Carbohydrate; 0mg Cholesterol; 5mg Sodium

Fruit Smoothie

What is cool and yummy and filling? Why it's a fruit smoothie. Try using your favorite fruit and enjoy!

6   ounces blueberries; fresh or frozen
4   ounces soft silken tofu or nonfat yogurt
2   tablespoons honey or to taste
1   cup ice
     fruit for garnish

Place all ingredients in blender. Blend on high speed until the texture is creamy and ice has been finely ground. Serve immediately.
Yield: 2 servings

🍎🍎🍎🍎🍎

Per serving: 119 Calories; 1g Fat (satfat 0g); 1g Protein; 30g Carbohydrate; 0mg Cholesterol; 9mg Sodium

Good Luck Punch

1   quart rhubarb cut 1 inch thick
     water
2   cups honey
6   each lemon juiced
1   cup pineapple juice
1   quart ginger ale

Cut rhubarb in 1" pieces; add water to cover. Cook until soft, about 10 minutes. Drain through cheesecloth bag or sugar sack. Measure - should be 3 quarts juice. Put honey and 2 cups water in pan and cook 10 minutes to make syrup. Add lemon, pineapple and rhubarb juices. Pour over chunk of ice in punch bowl. Just before serving add ginger ale or mineral water.
Yield: 1-gallon punch or 24 servings.

🍎🍎🍎🍎🍎

Per serving: 114 Calories; less than one gram Fat (satfat 0g); 1g Protein; 32g Carbohydrate; 0mg Cholesterol; 6mg Sodium

Hot Apple Punch

2 1/2   cups fructose or 1 1/2 c honey
4   cups water
2   each 2 1/2 inch cinnamon sticks
8   whole allspice berries
10   whole clove
1   whole ginger root
4   cups orange juice
2   cups lemon juice
2   quarts apple cider or apple juice

Combine fructose or honey and water and boil 5 minutes. Remove from heat; add spices. Let beverage stand, covered 1 hour. Strain. Just before serving, combine syrup, fruit juices and cider; bring quickly to boiling. Remove from heat: serve at once. *Yield: 27 servings*

🍎🍎🍎🍎🍎🍎

Per serving: 126 Calories; 1g Fat (satfat 0.2g); satfat 0.2; 1g Protein; 33g Carbohydrate; 0mg Cholesterol; 14mg Sodium

Island Sunset

2   each peaches, quartered
1/4   cup orange & pineapple juice, frozen concentrate
1   cup milk, fat free
1   teaspoon vanilla
3   each ice cubes, cracked

Combine peaches, milk, pineapple concentrate and vanilla in a blender or food processor. Whirl mixture until smooth. Add ice and swirl until smooth and fluffy.
Yield: 4 servings

🍎🍎🍎🍎🍎🍎

Per serving: 66 Calories; less than one gram Fat (satfat 0g); 3g Protein; 14g Carbohydrate; 1mg Cholesterol; 33mg Sodium

Old Fashioned Lemonade
I have never liked lemonade ... until now!
Donna, kitchen tester

4	each lemons
1/2	cup honey or Natural sugar*
1	quart water
1	tray ice cubes

Wash fruit. Cut into thin slices; remove seeds. Place lemon slices in a large bowl. Cover fruit with honey. Let stand 10 minutes, then press firmly with potato masher to extract juice. Add water; continue to press fruit with masher until liquid is well flavored. Add ice cubes. Taste lemonade for sweetness when it's chilled. Pour over two ice cubes in tall glasses; add lemon slices to each glass.
Yield: 7 glasses

Variations on a Theme
Lemon/Limeade: Use 2 limes and 2 lemons. Increase honey to 3/4 cup. Prepare according to directions for Old-Fashioned Lemonade.
Lemon/Orangeade: Use 2 oranges and 3 lemons. Decrease honey to 1/3 cup. Prepare according to directions for Old-Fashioned Lemonade.

Per serving: 86 Calories; less than one gram Fat (satfat 0g); 1g Protein; 27g Carbohydrate; 0mg Cholesterol; 7mg Sodium

Orange-Apricot Spritzer

2/3	cup orange juice
1/3	cup apricot nectar
1/2	cup club soda

Combine directly in each glass. Stir; set in refrigerator until time to serve; garnish with a sprig of mint.

Yield: 1 glass

Variations on a Theme
Instead of apricot juice use unsweetened pineapple juice, grapefruit juice, or any type of berry juice, a mild-flavored grape juice or any juices light in color. Garnish with thin slices of fresh apricot or orange or grated orange rind.

Per serving: 121 Calories; less than one gram Fat (satfat 0g); 1g Protein; 29g Carbohydrate; 0mg Cholesterol; 29mg Sodium

*my favorite is Florida Crystals Mill Cane Sugar

Plum Refresher

8	small plums, coarsely chopped
6	ounces cranberry cocktail, frozen concentrate
1	cup water

Combine all ingredients in blender or food processor. Whirl mixture until combined. *Yield: 8 servings*

🍎🍎🍎🍎🍎

Per serving: 55 Calories; less than one gram Fat (satfat 0g); 0g Protein; 14g Carbohydrate; 0mg Cholesterol; 2mg Sodium

Rhubarb Slush

3	cups rhubarb, chopped or frozen
1	cup water
1/3	cup natural sugar
1	cup apple juice
6	ounces pink lemonade, frozen concentrate, thawed
2	liters lemon-lime soda

In a saucepan, combine rhubarb, water and sugar; bring to a boil. Reduce heat; cover and simmer for 5 minutes or until rhubarb is tender. Cool for about 30 minutes. In a food processor or blender, puree mixture, half at a time. Stir in apple juice and lemonade. Pour into a freezer container; cover and freeze until firm. Let stand at room temperature for 45 minutes before serving. *Yield: 10 servings*

For individual servings, scoop 1/3 cup into a glass and fill with soda. To serve a group, place all of mixture in a large pitcher or punch bowl; add soda and stir. Serve immediately.

🍎🍎🍎🍎🍎

Per serving: 157 Calories; less than one gram Fat (satfat 0g); 0g Protein; 40g Carbohydrate; 0mg Cholesterol; 26mg Sodium

Tropical Slush

6	cups water, divided
5	medium bananas
1	cup fructose or natural sugar
24	ounces orange juice, frozen concentrate,thawed
12	ounces lemonade, frozen concentrate, thawed
46	ounces pineapple juice
6	liters lemon-lime soda

In a blender container, process 1-cup of water, bananas and fructose until smooth. Pour into a large container; add the concentrates, pineapple juice and remaining water. Cover and freeze. Remove from freezer 2 hours before serving. Just before serving, break up and mash mixture with a potato masher. Stir in soda.

Yield: 50 servings

🍎🍎🍎🍎🍎🍎

Per serving: 117 Calories; less than one gram Fat (satfat 0g); 1g Protein; 30g Carbohydrate; 0mg Cholesterol; 16mg Sodium

V-7 Juice

4	cups tomato juice
2	tablespoons lemon juice
2	stalks celery, chopped
1	teaspoon parsley, minced
1	tablespoon onion, minced
2	tablespoons green pepper, diced
1/4	teaspoon celery seed
	fresh ground pepper to taste

Combine 1 cup of tomato juice with lemon juice, celery, parsley, onion, green pepper and celery seed in blender. Blend at high speed until smooth. Add remaining juice and continue to blend until thoroughly mixed. Chill well before severing.

Yield: 5 1- cup servings.

🍎🍎🍎🍎🍎🍎

Per serving: 39 Calories; less than one gram Fat (satfat 0g); 2g Protein; 10g Carbohydrate; 0mg Cholesterol; 726mg Sodium

Very Berry Cooler

10	ounces strawberries, frozen
2	each peaches, cored and diced
12	each ice cubes, cracked/crushed

Combine frozen berries, peaches and ice in blender or food processor. Whirl until smooth.

Yield: *2 servings*

Variations on a Theme

Use 2 cups of fresh berries instead of frozen. Try raspberries or blueberries

🍎🍎🍎🍎🍎

Per serving: 139 Calories; less than one gram Fat (2% calories from fat); 1g Protein; 37g Carbohydrate; 0mg Cholesterol; 5mg Sodium

Apple-Cinnamon Granola

5	cups rolled oats *or* rolled wheat
1/2	cup cashews, finely chopped
1	cup coconut, flaked or shredded
1	teaspoon cinnamon
1/4	cup canola oil
1/2	cup wheat germ
1/2	cup honey or maple syrup
1 1/2	cups chopped dried fruit, evaporated
1	tablespoon brown sugar, firmly packed
1	teaspoon vanilla

Preheat oven to 250 F. Spread oats in an ungreased 13x9 baking pan and heat 10 minutes. Combine oats, coconut, cashews, wheat germ, and cinnamon in a large bowl. Stir in honey and oil and vanilla thoroughly. Mix until dry ingredients are well coated. Spoon into the same baking pan and bake 30 to 35 minutes stirring often to brown evenly. Toss apples in date sugar. Stir into granola until crumbly.

Yield: *16 servings*

🍎🍎🍎🍎🍎

Per serving: 228 Calories; 8g Fat (satfat 1.7g); 6g Protein; 35g Carbohydrate; 0mg Cholesterol; 5mg Sodium

Apple-Peach Granola

1/4	cup wheat germ
1/4	cup bran
1/4	cup rolled oats *or* rolled wheat
1/2	each apple, chopped
1/2	each peach, chopped
1	tablespoon shredded coconut
1	tablespoon sesame seeds

Combine all ingredients, tossing thoroughly. Can be served with milk or yogurt.
Yield: 2 servings

🍎🍎🍎🍎🍎🍎

Per serving: 168 Calories; 6g Fat (satfat 1.7g); 7g Protein; 27g Carbohydrate;
0mg Cholesterol; 12mg Sodium

Cashew Honey Butter

1	cup cashews, roasted
3	tablespoons margarine or soy margarine
2	tablespoons corn oil
1 1/2	tablespoons honey

Place all of the above ingredients in a blender until smooth. Put in refrigerator
and let set. Then add 2-3 tablespoons of margarine and beat in mixer. Put in
candy or butter molds, if desired and keep in refrigerator until ready for use.
Yield: 1 1/2 pounds (1 serving equals 2 tablespoons)

🍎🍎🍎🍎🍎🍎

Per serving: 116 Calories; 10g Fat (satfat 1.8g); 2g Protein; 5g Carbohydrate;
0mg Cholesterol; 35mg Sodium

Chili Seasoning Mix
Why buy chili mix from the store?
Now you can make it fresh and store it for later or use it right away!

1   tablespoon flour
2   tablespoons onion flakes
1 1/2   teaspoons chili powder
1   teaspoon seasoned salt
1/2   teaspoon red pepper, crushed dried
1/2   teaspoon garlic powder
1/2   teaspoon cumin powder

Combine all ingredients in a small bowl until evenly distributed. Spoon mixture onto a 6-inch square of aluminum foil and fold to make airtight. Label and date. Store in a cool, dry place.
Yield: 1 package (about 1/4 cup)

🌶🌶🌶🌶🌶

Per serving: 73 Calories; 1g Fat (satfat 0g); 2g Protein; 15g Carbohydrate; 0mg Cholesterol; 1408mg Sodium

Chinese Sauce

1 1/2   cups fat-free chicken broth *or* vegetarian broth
1   teaspoon molasses
1   teaspoon soy sauce
2   tablespoons cornstarch
2   tablespoons cold water

Combine chicken broth with molasses and soy sauce. Blend cornstarch and cold water add to chicken broth and cook, stirring constantly, over low heat until mixture comes to a boil.
Yield: about 1 1/2 cups.

🌶🌶🌶🌶🌶

Per serving: 18 Calories; 0g Fat (satfat 0g); 3g Protein; 4g Carbohydrate; 0mg Cholesterol; 176mg Sodium

Cranberry-Almond Cereal Mix

1	cup rolled oats
1	cup quick cooking barley
1	cup Bulgur *or* cracked wheat
1	cup cranberries, dried
1/2	cup sliced almonds, toasted
1	tablespoon cinnamon
1/4	teaspoon salt
	milk (optional)
	sweeten to taste

Up to six months ahead: In an airtight storage container stir together oats, barley, Bulgur or cracked wheat, cranberries or raisins, almonds, sugar, cinnamon and salt. Cover tightly; store in a cool, dry place for up to six months. Label and date.
For 1 serving: Stir mix. In a large microwave-safe cereal bowl, combine 3/4-cup water and 1/3 cup cereal mix. Cook, uncovered, on 50 percent power (medium) for 9 to 11 minutes or until cereal reaches desired consistency, stirring once during cooking. Stir before serving, if desired, serve with milk.
Yield: 7 servings

🍎🍎🍎🍎🍎

Per serving: 283 Calories; 7g Fat (satfat 0.8g); 9g Protein; 49g Carbohydrate; 0mg Cholesterol; 84mg Sodium

Fruit Slushy Mix

2	cups	honey
4	cups	water
6	ounces	orange juice, frozen concentrate
1/2	cup	lemon juice
46	ounces	pineapple juice

Combine honey and water in a medium saucepan. Heat until honey is dissolved. Add orange juice concentrate, lemon juice, and pineapple juice. Fill 6 or 7 ice cube trays with mixture. Freeze until firm. Remove ice cubes from freezer trays and store in plastic bags.
Yield: about 100 small cubes.

FRUIT SLUSH: Fill a glass with fruit slush cubes. Add ginger ale or Sparkling Mineral water and cover. Let stand 15 minutes. Stir and serve. Makes 1 serving.

🍎🍎🍎🍎🍎

Per serving: 193 Calories; 0g Fat (satfat 0g); 1g Protein; 51g Carbohydrate; 0mg Cholesterol; 5mg Sodium

Flax Seed Eggs

This works very well for binding, such as in burgers and loaves.

It also works well for cookies, quick breads, and cakes

2   **teaspoons flax seed flour***
3   **tablespoons water**

Place the ingredients in a small glass bowl or cup and microwave for 30 seconds on high. Remove and whisk with a fork until completely mixed. Refrigerate at least 15 minutes before using or until cool. When cooled mixture should have consistency of egg whites.
Yield: 1 egg or 2 egg whites

*To make flax seed flour, place flax seeds in blender and whirl until flour consistency. I find it is ultimately easier to grind an entire package of flax seeds and store in a tightly closed container so that I can use whenever I need to. If you make a lot of eggs at one time you can store them in the refrigerator in a jar for up to two weeks. Lable and date. 1/4 cup of mixture is equal to one egg or two egg whites.

🍎🍎🍎🍎🍎

Per serving: 19 Calories; 1g Fat (satfat 0.1g); 1g Protein; 1g Carbohydrate; 0mg Cholesterol; 4mg Sodium

Granola

4   **cups rolled oats**
1/2   **cup brown sugar, firmly packed**
1/3   **cup wheat germ**
1/3   **cup flaked or shredded coconut**
1/4   **cup sesame seeds**
1   **cup sliced almonds**
1/3   **cup honey *or* maple syrup**
1   **teaspoon vanilla**
1/4   **cup canola oil**

Heat oats in an ungreased 13x9-inch baking pan at 350 F. for 10 minutes. Combine oats, date sugar, wheat germ, coconut, sesame seeds and soybeans or almonds. Add oil, honey and vanilla; mix until dry ingredients are well coated. Bake in an ungreased 13x9-inch baking pan at 350 F. for 20 to 25 minutes, stirring often to brown evenly. Cool; stir until crumbly. Serve with cold milk, cream, or yogurt. Store in a tightly covered container in refrigerator.
Yield: 10 servings

🍎🍎🍎🍎🍎

Per serving: 359 Calories; 18g Fat (satfat 2.2g); 10g Protein; 43g Carbohydrate; 0mg Cholesterol; 8mg Sodium

Herbes de Provence

3	tablespoons marjoram, dried
3	tablespoons thyme, dried
3	tablespoons savory, dried
1	tablespoon basil, dried
1 1/2	teaspoons rosemary, dried and crumbled
1/2	teaspoon sage, dried
1/2	teaspoon fennel seed, optional

Combine herbs. Place in jar with a tight lid. To keep fresh for a long time store in refrigerator. Use any place you might use Italian seasoning. It is great with soups and sauces or over fresh vegetables.
Yield: about 2/3 cup

🍎🍎🍎🍎🍎

Per serving: 4 Calories; less than one gram Fat (satfat 0g); 0g Protein; 1g Carbohydrate; 0mg Cholesterol; 1mg Sodium

Season Salt

6	tablespoons sea salt
1/2	teaspoon celery seed
1/2	teaspoon marjoram
2 1/4	teaspoons paprika
1/4	teaspoon onion powder
1/8	teaspoon dill seed
1/2	teaspoon thyme
1/2	teaspoon garlic salt
1/2	teaspoon curry powder
1	teaspoon dry mustard

Mix all of the above ingredients together until evenly distributed. Place in and airtight container. Use wherever you want to spice things up. This is a good all around seasoning. *Yield: about 1/2 cup (serving size is a pinch)*

🍎🍎🍎🍎🍎

Per serving: 1 Calories; less than one gram Fat (satfat 0g); 0g Protein; 0g Carbohydrate; 0mg Cholesterol; 705mg Sodium

Appetizers, Beverages and So Forth

Seven Grain Mix

1	cup whole wheat flour
1	cup sunflower flour
1	cup wheat germ
1	cup oatmeal, ground
1	cup cornmeal
1	cup soy flour
1	cup rye flour

Combine and mix all ingredients. Measure one cup of mix into storage bags (should make 7 bags). Since most recipes call for 1 to 2 cups of flour, you won't even have to measure it out. This combination is always ready to use. It will bring superb nutrition to your breads, pancakes, muffins and cookies. Use wherever it calls for flour or other grain.
Yield: 7 cups

🍎🍎🍎🍎🍎

Per serving: 366 Calories; 6g Fat (satfat 0.7g); 20g Protein; 62g Carbohydrate; 0mg Cholesterol; 122mg Sodium

Super Salad Seasoning Mix

2	cups Kraft Free® nonfat grated topping *or* soy Parmesan cheese
2	teaspoons salt
1/2	cup sesame seeds
1/2	teaspoon garlic powder
1	tablespoon dried parsley
1/2	teaspoon dill seed
2	tablespoons poppy seeds
3	tablespoons celery seed
2	teaspoons paprika
1/2	teaspoon fresh ground pepper
1	tablespoon rosemary

Combine all ingredients in a small bowl. Mix until evenly distributed. Put in a 1-quart airtight container. Label. Store in a cool, dry place. Use within 3 to 4 months.
Yield: about 3 cups of Super Salad Seasoning Mix.

SUPER SALAD SEASONING MIX uses; Sprinkled topping over tossed green salads, baked potatoes, and buttered French bread or rolls, before toasting. Garnish for potato salads, macaroni or egg salads. Sour cream dip made with 2 tablespoons mix and 1 cup sour cream. Salad dressing made with 2 tablespoons mix and 1 cup salad dressing, mayonnaise, or yogurt.

🍎🍎🍎🍎🍎

Per serving: 25 Calories; 1g Fat (satfat 0.1g); 1g Protein; 3g Carbohydrate; 0mg Cholesterol; 124mg Sodium

Sweetened Condensed Milk

Make your own and know exactly what the ingredients are. Works just like the commercial version

4   cups powdered milk *or* soy milk powder
1   cup water   hot
1 1/2   cups honey *or* fructose *or* natural Sugar
1/4   cup margarine or soy margarine

Blend with mixer or put all the ingredients in a blender. Mix until sugar dissolves and store in the fridge.
Yield: 1 quart. 1 can equals 1 1/3 cups of this mixture. One serving is equal to 2 tablespoons.

🍎🍎🍎🍎🍎

Per serving: 136 Calories; 5g Fat (satfat 2.9); 4g Protein; 19g Carbohydrate; 16mg Cholesterol; 73mg Sodium

Taco Seasoning Mix

Why buy taco seasoning in the store when it so easy to make and you know that it is fresh?

2   tablespoons onion, minced instant
1   teaspoon sea salt
1   teaspoon chili powder
1/2   teaspoon cornstarch
1/2   teaspoon crushed red pepper
1/2   teaspoon garlic powder
1/2   teaspoon oregano
1/2   teaspoon cumin powder

Combine all ingredients in a small bowl until evenly distributed. Spoon mixture 9onto a 6-inch square of aluminum foil and fold to make airtight. Label. Store in a cool, dry place. Use within 6 months.
Yield: 1 package (about 2 tablespoons)

🍎🍎🍎🍎🍎

Per serving: 46 Calories; less than one gram Fat (satfat 0g); 0g Protein; 3g Carbohydrate; 0mg Cholesterol; 2160mg Sodium

Toasted Granola Surprise

2 1/2   cups wheat germ
2   cups rolled oats
1   cup bran
1   cup rye flakes *or* wheat flakes
1/2   cup walnuts, chopped *or* soynuts
1/2   cup sunflower seeds
1/2   cup sesame seeds
1/2   cup blackstrap molasses
1/2   cup honey
1/2   cup coconut flakes
1/2   cup canola oil

Mix all the ingredients until the molasses, honey and lecithin or oil is evenly distributed. Pour into a roasting pan or other large pan and toast it in the oven at 350 for 15 minutes or until the granola is somewhat dry and crispy. Stir occasionally for even browning. *Yield: 9 cups (serving size is 1/2 cup)*

Per serving: 278 Calories; 13g Fat (satfat 1.9g); 8g Protein; 37g Carbohydrate; 0mg Cholesterol; 15mg Sodium

Unflavored Gelatin Eggs

Here is another egg substitute that works well in desserts and baked goods

1   teaspoon gelatin
3   tablespoons cold water
1/2   cup boiling water

Place cold water in a mixing bowl and sprinkle gelatin in it to soften. Mix thoroughly. Add all the boiling water and stir until dissolved. Place mixture in freezer to thicken while preparing cake batter or other dessert ingredients. When recipe calls for an egg, take the mixture and whip it until it is frothy(like egg whites). Then add it to your batter. Works best to make and use gelatin eggs as you need them.
Yield: is equivalent to 1 egg or 2 egg whites.

Variations: To make 2 eggs use 2 teaspoons gelatin, 1/3 cup cold water and 1/2 cup boiling water.

Per serving: 3 Calories; less than one gram Fat (satfat 0g); 0g Protein; 0g Carbohydrate; 0mg Cholesterol; 6mg Sodium

Soups and Salads

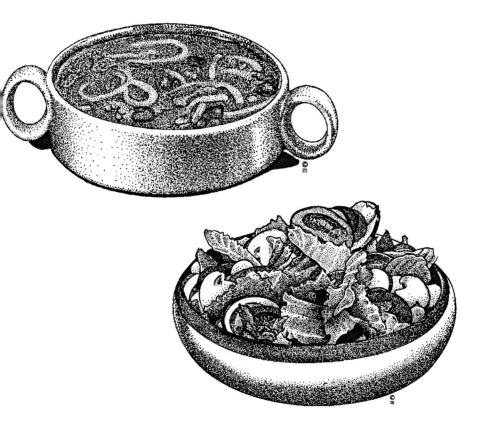

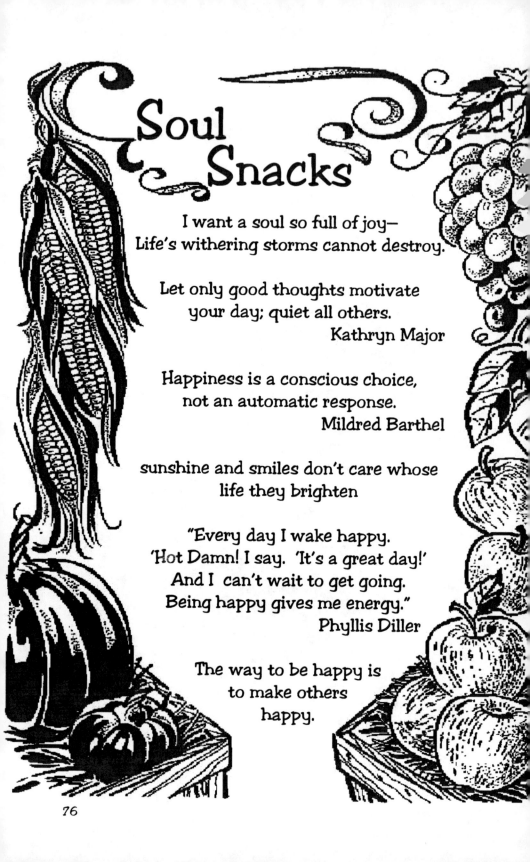

Soul Snacks

I want a soul so full of joy—
Life's withering storms cannot destroy.

Let only good thoughts motivate
your day; quiet all others.
Kathryn Major

Happiness is a conscious choice,
not an automatic response.
Mildred Barthel

sunshine and smiles don't care whose
life they brighten

"Every day I wake happy.
'Hot Damn! I say. 'It's a great day!'
And I can't wait to get going.
Being happy gives me energy."
Phyllis Diller

The way to be happy is
to make others
happy.

Ardy's Clam Chowder

2	cans clams, with liquid, minced
1	cup onions, finely chopped
1	cup celery, finely chopped
2	cups potatoes, finely diced
3/4	cup unbleached flour
4	cups evaporated skim milk or rice milk
1 1/2	teaspoons salt
	pepper to taste
1/2	teaspoon fructose or natural sugar
1/2	cup margarine or butter

Drain juice from clams and pour over vegetables in saucepan. Add enough water to barely cover and simmer covered over medium heat until potatoes are tender, about 20 minutes. In meantime melt margarine. Add flour to blend. Add milk, stirring until smooth and thick, using a wire whisk. Fold undrained vegetables and clams into milk mixture and heat through. Season with salt, pepper and fructose to taste.
Yield: 8 -10 servings

Personal Note: To enhance your individual serving my husband always adds a few drops of tabasco sauce.

🍎🍎🍎🍎🍎

Per serving: 230 Calories; 7g Fat (satfat 1.7g); 12g Protein; 27g Carbohydrate; 6mg Cholesterol; 861mg Sodium

Oriental Chicken and Vegetable Soup

4	pounds chicken breasts without skin
1	tablespoon oil
1 1/2	cups onions, chopped
1 1/2	cups carrots, chopped
1 1/2	cups celery, chopped
1	teaspoon curry powder
1	chopped Granny Smith apple
	salt and pepper to taste
2	cans fat-free chicken broth or vegetarian broth
10	ounces frozen corn
10	ounces frozen lima beans
1 1/2	cups cooked pasta shells
2	tablespoons fresh chopped parsley

In a 5-quart kettle or pot, pour oil and brown chicken until golden brown on all sides. Remove chicken and keep warm. In remaining oil in pan, saute onions, carrots, celery and curry powder. Use medium heat. Stir until onions are tender and limp; about 5 minutes.   Return chicken to pot. Add apple, salt, pepper, chicken broth, 5 cups cold water and parsley. Bring to a boil then reduce heat to simmer. Cover and simmer for 1 hour. Stir occasionally.

Remove chicken and bones from broth; cut chicken into bite-sized pieces. Add corn and lima beans and cook 15 minutes longer. Skim any additional fat from soup. Add pasta and return chicken to the pot. Cook another 10-15 minutes or until pasta is done.
Yield: 8-10 bowls of soup

🍎🍎🍎🍎🍎

Per serving: 318 Calories; 4g Fat (satfat 0.8g); 42g Protein; 30g Carbohydrate; 84mg Cholesterol; 346mg Sodium

Cheese and Broccoli Soup

1/3	cup onion, chopped
1	clove garlic, minced
1/3	cup celery, chopped
1	tablespoon olive oil
2	teaspoons Spike's All Purpose Seasoning®
2	teaspoons vegetarian bouillon
1/2	tablespoon parsley, dried
1	tablespoon basil leaves
1/2	teaspoon white pepper
1/2	teaspoon thyme
1 1/2	pounds broccoli
1 1/3	pounds potatoes, scrubbed & diced
	water
1/2	cup shredded lowfat cheddar cheese or soy cheddar cheese
1	cup shredded lowfat mozzarella cheese or soy cheese
1/3	cup skim milk *or* soy milk
5	cups water

In a stockpot or large saucepan, saute onions, garlic and celery in olive oil until tender. Turn heat to low and add all spices and herbs. Stir and let stand for one minute. Chop broccoli stems and leaves, reserving florets. Add chopped broccoli and diced potatoes to spice mixture. Cover with water and bring to a boil. Simmer mixture 20 minutes.

Break up and steam florets; set aside. Blend soup in a food processor until creamy. This may need to be done in batches. Return soup to pot. Add cheeses, milk, steamed florets. Heat mixture thoroughly but do no boil.
Yield: 10 bowls of soup

🍎🍎🍎🍎🍎

Per serving: 121 Calories; 4g Fat (satfat 1.7g); 8g Protein; 13g Carbohydrate; 7mg Cholesterol; 154mg Sodium

Appetizers, Beverages and So Forth

Chilled Fruit Soup

20	ounces frozen red raspberries, thawed
2	cups pineapple juice
1	tablespoon lime peel, grated
1	envelope unflavored gelatin
1/4	cup lime juice
2	tablespoons fructose or brown rice syrup

Carefully drain rasberries, reserving juice. Add water to juice to make 2 cups. In medium bowl, combine rasberry juice, rasberries, pineapple juice, and lime peel. In small cup, sprinkle gelatin over lime juice; let stand 5 minutes to soften. Set in pan of boiling water, stir until gelatin is dissolved. Stir into fruit-juice mixture, along with sugar. Refrigerate to chill well.
Yield: 6 bowls of soup

🍎🍎🍎🍎🍎

Per serving: 213 Calories; less than one gram Fat (satfat 0g); 2g Protein; 53g Carbohydrate; 0mg Cholesterol; 38mg Sodium

Cream of Mushroom Soup

2	quarts skim milk or rice milk
4	tablespoons margarine or soy margarine
4	tablespoons unbleached flour
4	cups evaporated skim milk or rice milk
1	tablespoon canola oil
1	pound sliced mushrooms
1	large onion, chopped fine
1	tablespoon garlic, chopped
1/2	teaspoon thyme
	salt and pepper

In a saucepan, cook milk slowly until it reduces in volume by half. Add 4 tablespoons margarine and 4 tablespoons flour and whisk until smooth. Add evaporated milk and bring just to a boil. In a small skillet melt butter and saute mushrooms and onions, stir into milk mixture. Whisk in garlic and thyme to milk mixture and cook briefly. Add salt and pepper to taste and mix well.
Yield: 8 bowls of soup

🍎🍎🍎🍎🍎

Per serving: 267 Calories; 6g Fat (satfat 1.4g); 20g Protein; 33g Carbohydrate; 9mg Cholesterol; 393mg Sodium

Creamy Tomato Soup

2	tablespoons flour
1	tablespoon fructose
2	cups evaporated skim milk *or* soy milk
4	cups tomato juice, heated
	fresh parsley, chopped

In a large saucepan, combine flour, sugar and 1/4 cup milk; stir until smooth. Add remaining milk. Bring to a boil over medium heat, stirring constantly. Cook and stir for 2 minutes or until thickened. Slowly stir in hot tomato juice until blended. Sprinkle with parsley.
Yield: 4 cups of soup

Variation on a Theme
For an herbed variation of this tasty soup use V-8 or V-7 juice (on page 64) instead of straight tomato juice.

🍎🍎🍎🍎🍎

Per serving: 163 Calories; less than one gram Fat (satfat 0.2g); 12g Protein; 30g Carbohydrate; 5mg Cholesterol; 1027mg Sodium

Easy Chili

1	16 oz-can kidney beans, drained
1	16 oz-can great northern beans, drained
1	16 oz-can pinto beans, drained
1	16 oz-can tomatoes with green chilis
1	16 oz-can tomato sauce
1	large green pepper, chopped
4	ounces chopped green chiles
1	large onion, chopped
3	cloves garlic, minced
2	tablespoons chili powder
1	tablespoon cumin powder
1	teaspoon basil
1	teaspoon oregano
2	dashes hot sauce
	pinchcrushed red pepper

Put all ingredients into a 5 quart saucepan and bring to a boil. Add spices, stir, cover partially and simmer 40 minutes.
Yield: 8 large bowls of chili

🍎🍎🍎🍎🍎

Per serving: 201 Calories; 1g Fat (satfat 0.2g); 12g Protein; 39g Carbohydrate; 0mg Cholesterol; 1096mg Sodium

French Onion Soup

4	cups onion, thinly sliced
1	clove garlic, minced
1/4	cup fat-free beef broth or vegetarian broth
6	cups water
8	cubes beef bouillon cubes or vegetarian bouillon
1	teaspoon Worcestershire sauce

In a large covered saucepan, cook onions and garlic in broth over medium-low heat for 8-10 minutes or until tender and golden, stirring occasionally. Add water, bouillon and Worcestershire sauce; bring to a boil. Reduce heat; cover and simmer for 30 minutes.
Yield: 6 bowls of soup

Variation on a Theme

If you want to present this soup in the classic French tradition ladle hot soup into six ovenproof bowls. (You will need 6 slices of french bread and 3 slices lowfat Swiss Cheese cut in half.) Top bowl with a piece of buttered and toasted French bread. Place a slice of cheese on bread. Broil until cheese melts. Serve immediately. (calories are now 200, total fat is 3.9g; and satfat 2.1g)

🍎🍎🍎🍎🍎

Per serving: 30 Calories; less than one gram of Fat (satfat 0.1g); 2g Protein; 5g Carbohydrate; 0mg Cholesterol; 1584mg Sodium

Italian Corn Chowder

1	large yellow onion, diced
2	stalks celery, diagonally sliced
1/4	cup fat-free chicken broth *or* vegetarian broth
2	pounds red potatoes, cubed
2	pounds frozen white corn
2	tablespoons fresh sage
2	tablespoons fennel seed
4	quarts evaporated skim milk or rice milk
4	cups water
	Salt and pepper

Saute onions and celery with butter in 5-quart stock pot. Add potatoes and corn, stir until mixed. Add milk and spices at the same time. Let soup come just to a boil, lower heat and add water. Simmer on low heat 45 minutes. Let stand 20 minutes at room temperature. Serve immediately.
Yield: 10 bowls of soup

🍎🍎🍎🍎🍎

Per serving: 459 Calories; 2g Fat (satfat 1.8g); 35g Protein; 79g Carbohydrate; 15mg Cholesterol; 496mg Sodium

Light Vegetable Soup With Tortellini

8	cups fat-free chicken broth or vegetarian broth
1	large onion, peeled and diced
2	large carrot, peeled and diced
2	stalks celery, diced
2	leeks, diced
2	zucchini, diced
1/2	teaspoon oregano
1/2	teaspoon basil
1	package frozen spinach-filled tortellini,
3	Roma tomato, chopped
	Salt and pepper
1/4	cup Kraft Free® nonfat grated topping or soy Parmesan cheese

Pour the broth into a large saucepan and add the onion, carrots, celery, leeks, zucchini and herbs. Simmer gently, covered, for 10 minutes to soften the vegetables. Add the tortellini and cook according to package directions or until al dente. The last 5 minutes of cooking add the chopped tomatoes. Season to taste .

Package in plastic containers and allow to cool, then refrigerate. Supply small packages of Parmesan cheese to sprinkle over the soup when served.
Yield: 8 bowls of soup

🍎🍎🍎🍎🍎

Per serving: 76 Calories; 1g Fat (satfat 0.4g); 14g Protein; 12g Carbohydrate; 16mg Cholesterol; 634mg Sodium

Fill'er Up Soup

I found this recipe in a really old book when I was a teenager it was called Mormon Whole Meal Soup. When I was growing up my brothers would often be heard to say, "My bowls Empty ... Fill'er up!" so I have renamed it after them.

2	quartswater
12	ouncesMorningstar® Harvest Burgers Recipe Crumbles
	or 1 1/2 pounds extra lean ground beef
1	cup celery,diced
1	cup corn
2	cups cabbage, shredded
1 1/2	teaspoons salt
2	cups potatoes, diced
2	cups tomatoes, stewed
1	cup carrots, diced
2	onion, diced
1/4	cup rice

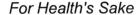

For Health's Sake

In a large stock pot add water and crumbles, bring to a roiling boil. Add cut celery, corn, potatoes, tomatoes, carrot, onion and return to a boil. Add rice and cabbage and season to taste. Simmer for 1 to 1 1/2 hours. Makes a large hearty pot of soup. (*If you use extra lean ground beef the calories are 187, total fat 10g and satfat 3.9g)
Yield: 10-12 bowls of hearty soup

Personal Note: If you want to come home to a wonderfully heart warming soup on a cold evening. Place all the ingredients into a large crockpot and let it simmer all day on low. Then when you get home bake up a fresh batch of corn meal muffins and enjoy an easy light supper.

🍎🍎🍎🍎🍎🍎

Per serving: 45 Calories; less than one gram Fat (satfat 0.1); 2g Protein; 9g Carbohydrate; 0mg Cholesterol; 288mg Sodium

Potato Chowder

4	large potatoes
3	tablespoons fat-free chicken broth
1/4	cup green onions, diced
1/2	cup green pepper, diced
2	cups water
1	teaspoon salt
1/8	teaspoon pepper
1/4	teaspoon paprika
3	tablespoons unbleached flour
2	cups evaporated skim milk *or* soy milk
1	can corn *or* 1 cup frozen corn
1/2	cup celery chopped

Peel and dice potatoes. In large saucepan saute onions, green pepper and celery. Cook until tender. Add potatoes, water and seasonings. Cover and simmer until potatoes are tender. Make paste of flour and 1/3 cup of water. Add milk and cook until slightly thickened. Stir in undrained corn. Heat thoroughly and serve.
Yield: 10 bowls of soup

🍎🍎🍎🍎🍎🍎

Per serving: 86 Calories; less than one gram Fat (satfat 0.1); 5g Protein; 16g Carbohydrate; 2mg Cholesterol; 322mg Sodium

Appetizers, Beverages and So Forth

Potato-Cheese Soup

3	medium potatoes, cut up
1	small onion, diced
3	tablespoons fat-free chicken broth or vegetarian broth
2	cups skim milk or soy milk
2	tablespoons flour
2	tablespoons parsley, snipped
3/4	teaspoon salt
	dash pepper
1	cup shredded lowfat Swiss cheese *or* soy mozarrela cheese

In a 2 quart saucepan add potatoes and onion to 1 cup lightly salted boiling water. Cover and cook about 20 minutes, or until potatoes are tender. Mash potatoes slightly; do not drain. Measure mixture and add enough milk to make 5 cups. Blend broth, flour, parsley, salt, and pepper together until smooth. Stir into potato mix in saucepan, cook and stir till thickened and bubbly. Add cheese, cook and stir until cheese is partially melted. Serve immediately.
Yield: 6 bowls of soup

🍎🍎🍎🍎🍎🍎

Per serving: 114 Calories; 1g Fat (satfat 0.7g); 10g Protein; 16g Carbohydrate; 8mg Cholesterol; 474mg Sodium

Apple Salad

8		apples, chopped
1/2	cup	celery, diced
1/2	cup	dates, chopped
1/2	cup	nuts, chopped
2	tablespoons	lemon juice
		Salad dressing or whipped topping, optional

Combine apples, celery, dates, nuts, and lemon juice. Toss and chill. Serve on lettuce leaf, with a dollop of salad dressing or whipped topping, if desired.
Yield: 10 servings

🍎🍎🍎🍎🍎🍎

Per serving: 127 Calories; 4g Fat (satfat 0.7g); 2g Protein; 23g Carbohydrate; 0mg Cholesterol; 6mg Sodium

Almond Citrus Salad

1/3	cup orange juice
2	tablespoons white wine vinegar or apple cider vinegar
2	tablespoons canola oil
1	tablespoon honey
2	teaspoons fresh ginger, grated
1/4	teaspoon salt
1/8	teaspoon red pepper flakes
2	large grapefruit, peeled & segmented
2	large navel oranges, peeled and sliced
1/4	cup red onion, finely chopped
6	cups spinach leaves, torn into bite size pieces
1/3	cup slivered almonds, toasted

To make dressing, in container of blender combine juice, vinegar, oil, honey, ginger, salt and pepper flakes. Blend to mix thoroughly. In bowl combine fruit, onion and dressing. Set aside for at least 10 minutes or up to 1 hour.

To serve, line four individual plates with spinach. Spoon fruit mixture with dressing over spinach, dividing equally. Sprinkle almonds over salads.
Yield: 4 servings

🍎🍎🍎🍎🍎🍎

Per serving: 234 Calories; 14g Fat (satfat 1.1g); 6g Protein; 27g Carbohydrate; 0mg Cholesterol; 183mg Sodium

Cabbage and Pineapple Salad

2	cups	shredded cabbage
4	slices	pineapple
1/4	cup	peanuts, chopped
1/3	cup	Miracle Whip® light

Combine cabbage, diced fruit, and nuts. Mix with salad dressing. Serve on lettuce or in tomato cups. Apple may be used for the pineapple.
Yield: 6 servings

🍎🍎🍎🍎🍎🍎

Per serving: 340 Calories; 9g Fat (satfat 0.6g); 4g Protein; 70g Carbohydrate; 3mg Cholesterol; 95mg Sodium

Ambrosia Platter

1	large pineapple
2	large oranges
2	large bananas
1	tablespoon lemon juice
	shredded coconut
3	strawberries, stem removed

Cut off pineapple top. With a sharp knife, cut pineapple into slices 1/2-inch thick. Remove core with a 1 1/2-inch round cookie cutter. With knife remove rind (including eyes) from each slice. With sharp knife remove peel from oranges; cut into slices 1/3-inch thick. Peel bananas; slice on diagonal into 2-inch pieces. Toss with lemon juice.

On serving platter, place an orange slice in center of each pineapple slice. Arrange around edge of platter, overlapping. Turn bananas into center; sprinkle all over with a little orange juice if desired. Sprinkle coconut over top. Slice strawberries; garnish platter. Refrigerate to chill, before serving.
Yield: 8 servings

🍎🍎🍎🍎🍎🍎

Per serving: 95 Calories; 1g Fat (satfat 0.1g); 1g Protein; 26g Carbohydrate; 0mg Cholesterol; 2mg Sodium

Cranberry Blizzard
Especially good when served with chicken or turkey.

1	pound whole cranberries
2	cups water
1	cup fructose or natural sugar
2	tablespoons unflavored gelatin
1/2	cup cold water
1	cup lowfat cottage cheese

Boil together cranberries and 2 cups water, 5 minutes. Add sugar and boil 5 more minutes. Soften gelatin in 1/2-cup cold water. Dissolve gelatin in hot cranberries. Cool and pour into 8" ring mold. Chill overnight. Unfold on lettuce leaves. Fill center with cottage cheese.
Yield: 10 servings

🍎🍎🍎🍎🍎🍎

Per serving: 90 Calories; less than one gram Fat (satfat 0.1g); 3g Protein; 21g Carbohydrate; 1mg Cholesterol; 87mg Sodium

French Tomato Salad

4	large tomatoes, sliced
4	tablespoons canola oil
4	tablespoonswine vinegar *or* apple cider vinegar
1	onion, sliced in rings
1	teaspoon Herbes de Provence *or* Italian Seasoning
	salt and pepper

Cut tomatoes into slices. Arrange on a plate with the onion slices. Mix oil, vinegar and herbs together. Pour the oil and vinegar mixture over the tomatoes and onions and then sprinkle the whole dish with the herbs and salt and pepper. Cover and refrigerate until ready to serve.
Yield: 8 servings

Variation on a Theme
Add 1 sliced cucumber before you cover in oil and vinegar.

🍎🍎🍎🍎🍎

Per serving: 78 Calories; 7g Fat (satfat 0.5g); 1g Protein; 4g Carbohydrate; 0mg Cholesterol; 74mg Sodium

Hot German Potato

1	tablespoon oil
4	green onions, sliced thin
1	tablespoon unbleached flour
1	tablespoon fructose or natural sugar
1	tablespoon parsley
2	tablespoons Dijon mustard
1/2	teaspoon salt
1/2	teaspoon pepper
4	cups potatoes, sliced
1/4	cup apple cider vinegar

Heat oil in large skillet. Add green onions to hot oil and sauté until tender. Stir in flour, sugar, parsley, mustard, salt and pepper. Gradually add 1/2 cup reserved potato water, and the vinegar. Cook and stir until mixture thickens and boils. Stir in cooked potato slices and heat through.
Yield: 4-6 servings

🍎🍎🍎🍎🍎

Per serving: 148 Calories; 4g Fat (satfat 0.5g); 5g Protein; 27g Carbohydrate; 0mg Cholesterol; 392mg Sodium

Fruit Salad with Orange Poppy Seed Dressing

Soups and Salads

1/2	cup orange juice
3	tablespoons cider vinegar
3	tablespoons mustard
2	tablespoons honey
2	tablespoons Worcestershire sauce
1	teaspoon grated orange peel
1/2	teaspoon salt
1	tablespoon cornstarch *or* arrowroot
1/2	cup water
1	tablespoon poppy seeds
1	cup orange, sliced
1	cup cantaloupe, sliced
1	cup watermelon, sliced
1	cup grapes
1	cup blueberries
1	cup honeydew melon, sliced
	lettuce leaves

In small saucepan mix cornstarch and water. Heat to just below the boiling point while beating with an eggbeater or whisk. After it thickens, set aside to cool while you prepare the rest of the ingredients. Now place juice, vinegar, mustard, honey, Worcestershire, orange peel and salt in blender or food processor. Cover and process until well blended. Add slightly cooled cornstarch, processing until very smooth. Stir in poppy seeds. Chill until ready to serve.

Arrange fruit on lettuce leaves on large platter. Spoon dressing over fruit just before serving.
Yield: 6-8 servings

Per serving: 108 Calories; 1g Fat (satfat 0.1g); 2g Protein; 25g Carbohydrate; 0mg Cholesterol; 333mg Sodium

Light and Fruity Salad

2	cups fat-free whipped topping
1	cup lowfat cottage cheese
1	cup crushed pineapple in juice, drained
1	cup strawberries, sliced
3	ounces strawberry gelatin powder

Mix cottage cheese, drained pineapple, strawberries together in medium sized bowl. Fold in whipped topping and gelatin until smooth. Chill till ready to serve.
Yield: 5 cups (serving size 1/2 cup)

Variations on a Theme
Try blueberries with wild berry gelatin or one of our favorites is mandarin oranges, drained with orange or apricot gelatin. The combinations are endless, by just changing the strawberries for another fruit and choosing a complimentary gelatin. You can also add sliced almonds for a festive touch.

🍎🍎🍎🍎🍎

Per serving: 92 Calories; less than one gram Fat (satfat 0.1g); 4g Protein; 18g Carbohydrate; 1mg Cholesterol; 130mg Sodium

Mouthwatering Fruit Salad

1	cup pineapple chunks in juice, drained
1	cup fresh peaches, diced
1	cup seedless grapes
1	cup melon balls
1	large bananas, sliced
2	large pears, diced
1	large apples, diced
	other fresh fruit as desired
2	cups fat-free whipped topping
1	cup nonfat apricot/pineapple yogurt
1	tablespoon honey

Prepare fruits as instructed above (use amounts of each as you desire), and mix together and chill. Then whip cream till it is stiff. Toss together whipped cream, yogurt, honey, and all the prepared fruit. Keep chilled till ready to serve. Makes as much as you mix together.
Yield: 8 servings

🍎🍎🍎🍎🍎

Per serving: 150 Calories; less than one gram Fat (satfat 0.1g); 2g Protein; 36g Carbohydrate; 1mg Cholesterol; 46mg Sodium

Norwegian Fruit Salad

2	oranges
1	small banana
3/4	cup grapes
1/4	cup walnuts or sliced almonds
1	small red delicious apples
1	teaspoon lemon juice
1	teaspoon water
1 1/2	cups Lemon fruit salad dressing (see page)

Peel oranges and separate into sections. Peel banana; coarsely chop. Cut grapes in half. Chop walnuts, cut apple in quarters, core, and then chop coarsely; sprinkle with diluted lemon juice. Combine fruits, walnuts, then refrigerate. Serve lemon fruit salad dressing over chilled fruit mix.
Yield: 6 servings

🍎🍎🍎🍎🍎

Per serving: 70 Calories; 1g Fat (satfat 0.1g); 1g Protein; 18g Carbohydrate; 0mg Cholesterol; 4mg Sodium

Orange Cream Fruit Salad

20	ounces pineapple tidbits in juice, drained
16	ounces peach slices, drained
1	11 oz-can mandarin oranges, drained
2	medium bananas, sliced
1	medium apple, chopped
1	3 oz-pkg. vanilla instant pudding mix
1 1/2	cups skim milk
1/3	cup orange juice, frozen concentrate
3/4	cup sour cream, light

In a large salad bowl, combine fruits; set aside. In a small mixing bowl, beat pudding mix, milk and orange juice concentrate for 2 minutes. Add sour cream; mix well. Spoon over fruit; toss to coat. Cover and refrigerate for 2 hours.
Yield: 8 servings

🍎🍎🍎🍎🍎

Per serving: 181 Calories; 1g Fat (satfat 0.1g); 3g Protein; 43g Carbohydrate; 3mg Cholesterol; 127mg Sodium

Raw Cauliflower Salad

1	small cauliflower, thinly sliced
3	red delicious apples, diced
1	cup celery, sliced
3	small green onion, sliced
3/4	cup parsley, chopped
1	clove garlic
1/2	teaspoon salt
1/4	cup red wine vinegar *or* apple cider vinegar
1/4	cup plain nonfat yogurt *or* soy yogurt
	pepper to taste

Thoroughly chill prepared cauliflower, apples, celery, onions and parsley in a plastic bag. Rub salad bowl with cut garlic clove and salt. Shake vinegar, yogurt and pepper vigorously in a tightly covered jar. Pour over mixed fruit and vegetables; toss lightly.
Yield: 6 servings

Per serving: 93 Calories; 1g Fat (satfat 0.1g); 4g Protein; 21g Carbohydrate; 0mg Cholesterol; 248mg Sodium

Salmon Salad Sandwich

2/3	cup canned salmon, flaked
1/2	medium cucumber, diced 1/4" cubes
5	tablespoons plain nonfat yogurt
1	teaspoon lemon juice
2	teaspoons onion, finely minced
1	teaspoon chives, chopped
1	piece whole wheat pita bread, halved

Combine all ingredients except bread. Chill. Serve in pita pockets. (Tuna or chicken may be used in place of salmon.)
Yield: 2 sandwiches

Per serving: 225 Calories; 6g Fat (satfat 1.4g); 21g Protein; 23g Carbohydrate; 44mg Cholesterol; 648mg Sodium

Three Bean Salad

1	can green beans, drained
1	can wax beans, drained
1	can kidney beans, drained
1	medium onion, sliced
1	large cucumber, sliced
1/2	cup fructose or natural sugar
1/3	cup vinegar, cider
	salt and pepper

Put all the beans into a bowl or large glass jar. Add sliced cucumbers and onions. Mix together fructose, vinegar and salt and pepper. Toss all together and let set in refrigerator all night before serving. The longer it sets the better it gets.
Yield: 8 servings

Personal Note: I always add extra cucumbers they are just so tasty.

🍎🍎🍎🍎🍎

Per serving: 130 Calories; less than one gram Fat (satfat 0.1g); 6g Protein; 28g Carbohydrate; 0mg Cholesterol; 78mg Sodium

Tropical Fruit Mold

3	envelopes	unflavored gelatin
16	ounce, can	pear halves
2	cups	grapefruit juice, unsweetened
2	cups	pineapple juice
1	cup	grapefruit sections
1	cup	honeydew melon balls
1	cup	cantaloupe balls

In medium saucepan, sprinkle gelatin over 1/2 cup water; let stand 5 minutes to soften. Drain pears; reserve liquid (1 cup). Place gelatin over medium heat; stir until gelatin is dissolved; remove from heat. Add reserved pear juice, grapefruit and pineapple juices; mix well. Set bowl with gelatin in bowl containing ice water, stirring occasionally, until mixture is consistency of unbeaten egg whites - 15 to 20 minutes. Turn into 5-cup decorative mold. Refrigerate until firm - 3 to 4 hours or overnight. Unmold onto large platter. Arrange grapefruit sections, melon balls, and grapes around mold.
Yield: 8-10 servings

🍎🍎🍎🍎🍎

Per serving: 225 Calories; less than one gram Fat (satfat 0g); 4g Protein; 54g Carbohydrate; 0mg Cholesterol; 86mg Sodium

Tahitian Salad

5	medium carrot, finely shredded
1	cup crushed pineapple
1	cup shredded coconut
	pinch salt

Mix all ingredients. Salad may be served with a salad dressing, if desired.
Yield: 5 servings

Per serving: 68 Calories; 3g Fat (satfat 2.5); 1g Protein; 10g Carbohydrate;
0mg Cholesterol; 27mg Sodium

Tico Taco Salad

1/2	pound extra lean ground beef, browned and drained *or* Morningstar® Harvest Burger Recipe Crumbles
15	ounces kidney beans, drained
2	medium tomatoes, chopped
1	medium onion, chopped
1	package Taco seasoning mix (see page)
10	ounces baked tortilla chips, crumbled
1	cup shredded lowfat cheddar cheese
1	head lettuce, torn into bite size pieces.
	salsa
	sour cream, light

Fry beef and add seasoning. Drain beans and rinse well. Combine all ingredients; toss well. Serve immediately.
Yield: 6 servings

Variation on a Theme
For a tasty change serve with guacamole in your own tortilla bowl. To make
tortilla bowl: spray a glass or metal bowl with vegetable spray and lay a flour
tortilla over bowl. Spray outside of tortilla with a light coat of vegetable spray.
Then place in a 350°F oven for about 5 minutes or until slightly golden and
baked. Then fill your own tortilla bowl with you Tico Taco Salad

Per serving: 590 Calories; 10g Fat (satfat 3.6g); 33g Protein; 86g Carbohydrate;
30mg Cholesterol; 738mg Sodium

Soups and Salads

Vitamin-Carrot Salad

2	cups carrots, grated
2	tablespoons lemon juice
1	cup celery, diced
1/4	cup walnuts, finely chopped
1/4	cup plain nonfat yogurt

In a medium sized bowl place carrots, celery and walnuts. Cream together lemon juice and yogurt. Lightly toss all ingredients with dressing. Chill. Serve on salad greens.
Yield: 6 servings

🍎🍎🍎🍎🍎

Per serving: 31 Calories; 1g Fat (satfat 0.1g); 1g Protein; 5g Carbohydrate; 0mg Cholesterol; 34mg Sodium

Zucchini Toss

	Olive oil spray
1	head lettuce, washed & chilled
1	bunch romaine lettuce, washed & chilled
2	medium zucchini, thinly sliced
1	cup radishes, sliced
3	green onions, sliced
2	tablespoons blue cheese, crumbled
2	tablespoons wine vinegar *or* apple cider vinegar
1/2	teaspoon salt
1	clove garlic, crushed
	pepper to taste

Into a large salad bowl, tear greens into bite-sized pieces. Spray greens with olive oil spray and toss with oil until leaves glisten. Add zucchini, radishes, onions and cheese. Combine vinegar, salt, garlic, and pepper; pour over salad mixture and toss.
Yield: 6 servings

🍎🍎🍎🍎🍎

Per serving: 65 Calories; 1g Fat (satfat 0.5g); 5g Protein; 12g Carbohydrate; 2mg Cholesterol; 240mg Sodium

Breads

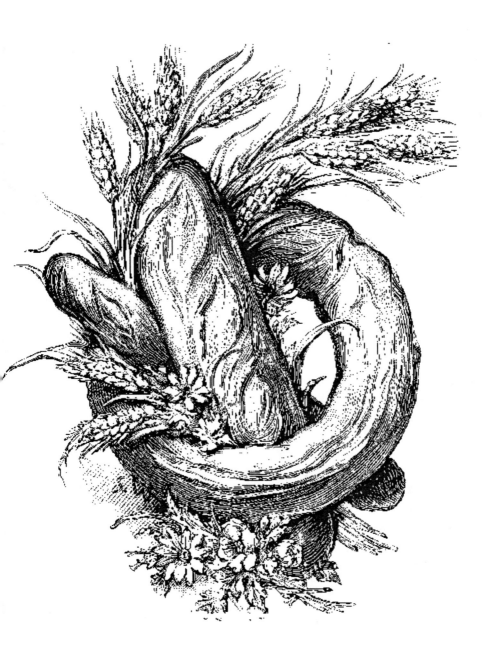

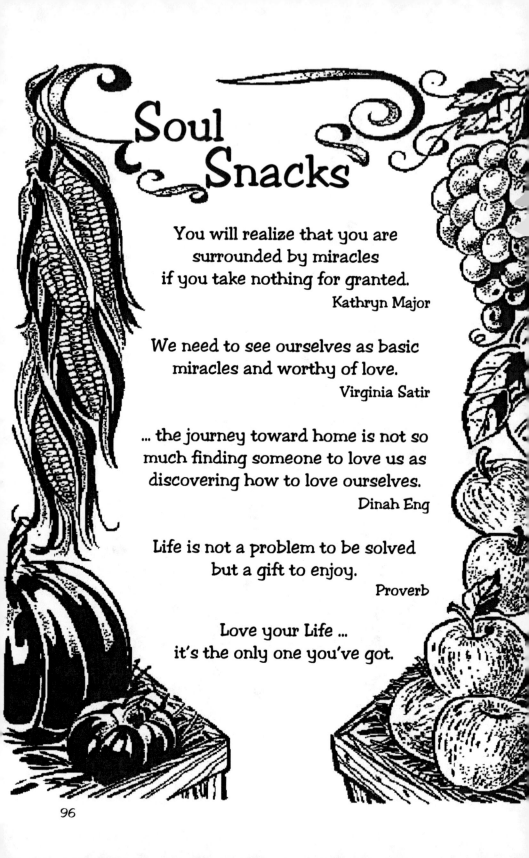

Soul Snacks

You will realize that you are
surrounded by miracles
if you take nothing for granted.

Kathryn Major

We need to see ourselves as basic
miracles and worthy of love.

Virginia Satir

... the journey toward home is not so
much finding someone to love us as
discovering how to love ourselves.

Dinah Eng

Life is not a problem to be solved
but a gift to enjoy.

Proverb

Love your Life ...
it's the only one you've got.

Apple Bran Muffins

2	large golden delicious apples, peeled & chopped
1/2	cup apple juice
3	cups All-Bran® Cereal
1	cup boiling water
1 3/4	cups buttermilk *or* soy milk + lemon juice
3	egg whites *or* 1/4 cup tofu
1/2	cup honey
1	cup raisins
2 1/2	cups unbleached flour
2 1/2	teaspoons baking soda
2	teaspoons cinnamon
1	teaspoon nutmeg
1/2	teaspoon cloves
1/2	teaspoon salt

In a skillet, sauté apples in apple juice until tender, about 10 minutes. Combine cereal and water in a large bowl; stir in the buttermilk, eggs, sugar, raisins and apples with juice. Combine dry ingredients; stir into apple mixture just until moistened. Refrigerate in a tightly covered container for at least 24 hours (batter will be very thick). Fill greased or paper-lined muffin cups three-fourths full. Bake at 400 for 20-25 minutes or until muffins test done. Cool in pan 10 minutes before removing to a wire rack.
Yield: 24 muffins

Note: Batter can be stored in a tightly covered container in the refrigerator for up to 2 weeks.

🍎🍎🍎🍎🍎🍎

Per serving: 131 Calories; 1g Fat (satfat 0.2); 4g Protein; 31g Carbohydrate; 1mg Cholesterol; 325mg Sodium

For Health's Sake

Berry Cream Muffins

4	cups unbleached flour
1 1/2	cups fructose or natural sugar
2	teaspoons baking powder
1	teaspoon baking soda
1/4	teaspoon salt
3	cups raspberries, frozen or fresh
2	eggs, lightly beaten
4	egg whites
1 1/2	cups light sour cream
1	cup unsweetened applesauce
1	teaspoon vanilla extract

In a large bowl, combine flour, sugar, baking powder, baking soda and salt; add berries and toss gently. Combine eggs, sour cream, oil and vanilla; mix well. Stir into dry ingredients just until moistened. Fill greased or paper-lined muffin cups two-thirds full. Bake at 400 for 20-25 minutes or until muffins test done.

Yield: 24 muffins

🍎🍎🍎🍎🍎

Per serving: 162 Calories; 1g Fat (satfat 0.1g); 4g Protein; 35g Carbohydrate; 16mg Cholesterol; 124mg Sodium

Dilly Cheddar Muffins

3 1/2	cups unbleached flour
2	tablespoons fructose or natural sugar
2	tablespoons baking powder
2	teaspoons dill weed
1	teaspoon salt
2/3	cup shredded lowfat cheddar cheese or soy cheddar cheese
1 1/2	cups skim milk or soy milk
2	flax seed eggs or 2 egg whites + 1 egg
1/4	cup canola oil

In a bowl, combine the first six ingredients. Combine milk, eggs and butter; stir into dry ingredients just until moistened. Fill greased or paper-lined muffin cups almost full. Bake at 400 for 25-30 minutes or until muffins test done. Cool in pan 10 minutes before removing to a wire rack.

Yield: 12 muffin

🍎🍎🍎🍎🍎

Per serving: 208 Calories; 5.4g Fat (satfat 0.7g); 7g Protein; 31g Carbohydrate; 2mg Cholesterol; 415mg Sodium

Golden Corn Muffins

1	cup yellow cornmeal
1	cup unbleached flour
1/4	cup honey
4	teaspoons baking powder
1/2	teaspoon salt
3	egg whites or 2 eggs
3/4	cup buttermilk *or* yogurt
1/4	cup canola oil

Sift together corn meal, flour, honey, baking powder, and salt. Add eggs, milk, and oil. Beat with a fork until all ingredients are moistened. Grease muffin tins. Fill muffin tins 2/3 full. Bake in preheated oven, 425 degrees 15-20 minutes. *Yield: 12 muffins*

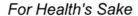

Per serving: 147 Calories; 5g Fat (satfat 0.5g) 3g Protein; 23g Carbohydrate; 1mg Cholesterol; 244mg Sodium

Good Morning Muffins

2	cups pineapple juice, lukewarm
2	cups golden raisins
1	cup brown sugar packed
1/2	cup vegetable oil
1/2	cup honey
5	flax seed eggs or eggs
2	cups all-purpose flour
2	teaspoons baking soda
1	teaspoon salt
4	cups All-Bran® Cereal

In a small bowl, combine pineapple juice and raisins; set aside. In a large mixing bowl, combine brown sugar, oil, honey and eggs; mix well. Combine flour, baking soda and salt; stir in cereal. Add to sugar mixture and mix well. Fold in the raisin mixture (batter will be thin). Cover and refrigerate at least 3 hours or overnight. Stir (batter will thicken). Fill greased or paper-lined muffin cups three-fourths full. Bake at 400 for 20-25 minutes or until muffins test done. Cool in pan 10 minutes before removing to a wire rack. *Yield: 20 muffins*

Per serving: 247 Calories; 6g Fat (satfat 0.7g); 4g Protein; 51g Carbohydrate; 0mg Cholesterol; 432mg Sodium

Golden Raisin Buns

2   **cups hot water, divided**
1/2   **cup golden raisins**
1/2   **cup margarine**
1   **teaspoon fructose or natural sugar**
1/4   **teaspoon salt**
1   **cup unbleached flour**
2   **eggs**
3   **egg whites**
                 ICING
1   **tablespoon margarine**
4   **teaspoons evaporated skim milk *or* soy milk**
1   **cup confectioner's sugar**
1/2   **teaspoon lemon juice**
1/2   **teaspoon vanilla extract**

In a small bowl, pour 1 cup of water over raisins; let stand for 5 minutes. Drain; set raisins aside. In a large saucepan, bring 1/2-cup butter, sugar, salt and remaining water to a boil. Add flour all at once; stir until smooth ball forms. Remove from the heat; beat by hand for 2 minutes. Add eggs, one at a time, beating well after each addition. Beat until mixture is well blended, about 3 minutes. Stir in the raisins. Drop by tablespoonfuls 2 in. apart onto greased baking sheets. Bake at 375 for 30-35 minutes or until golden brown. Transfer to a wire rack. For icing, melt 1-tablespoon butter in a small saucepan; stir in milk. Remove from the heat; add confectioners' sugar, lemon juice and vanilla. Spread on buns while still warm. Serve warm if desired.

Yield: 20 buns

🍎🍎🍎🍎🍎

Per serving: 99 Calories; 4g Fat (satfat 0.7g); 2g Protein; 14g Carbohydrate; 18mg Cholesterol; 88mg Sodium

Honey Graham Crackers

1	cup unbleached flour
2	cups whole wheat flour
1/2	teaspoon baking soda
1	teaspoon baking powder
1/4	teaspoon salt
1/2	cup margarine
1/4	cup honey
1/3	cup brown sugar
1/2	cup skim milk
1/2	teaspoon cinnamon

Sift flours together with baking powder, baking soda, salt and cinnamon. Add margarine, vanilla, fructose, and honey and mix, alternate with milk. Knead dough a dozen times. Divide dough into 4 balls and roll each into a log. Wrap in plastic wrap and chill one hour (can be chilled overnight). Roll out one log 15x15-inches (hint the thinner the cracker the crisper it is) about 1/4 - 1/2 inches thick. Then using a pizza wheel cut dough into 2-inch squares, poke each square a few times with the tines of a fork. Place squares on a cookie sheet. Bake at 350°F for 12-14 minutes. Continue rolling and cutting dough till all crackers are baked. Keep in an airtight container.
Yields: about 100 graham cracker squares.

Variations on a Theme
For fun you can dust these crackers with a cinnamon-sugar mixture before you bake them. Also try using oat flour in place of the whole-wheat flour.

I also find that this a great replacement for the traditional graham cracker crust. You can roll it out just like a regular piecrust, bake it and fill it just like a regular graham cracker crust.

🍎🍎🍎🍎🍎

Per serving: 23 Calories; 1g Fat (satfat 0.1g); 1g Protein; 4g Carbohydrate; 0mg Cholesterol; 24mg Sodium

Morning Glory Breakfast Muffins

If you want to reduce the fat even more eliminate the sunflower seeds (a source of good fats) and your total fat is 2.6g (satfat 0.2g) and calories 115.

2/3	cup sunflower seeds, roasted
3/4	cup whole wheat flour
3/4	cup all-purpose flour
1	teaspoon baking powder
1/2	teaspoon baking soda
1/2	teaspoon salt
1	teaspoon cinnamon
1	egg
2	tablespoons canola oil
3/4	cup carrots, grated
1/2	cup unsweetened applesauce
1/2	cup dark brown sugar, packed
1/2	cup orange juice
1	teaspoon vanilla extract
1/2	cup raisins

Heat oven to 375° F. Lightly coat 12 muffin cups with vegetable oil spray or line with paper liners. Whisk together sunflower seeds, whole-wheat and white flours, baking powder, baking soda, salt and cinnamon. Whisk egg with oil until smooth. Add grated carrot, applesauce, brown sugar, orange juice and vanilla and whisk until blended. Stir in raisins.

Add carrot mixture to flour mixture. Whisk until just combined. Do not overtax. Spoon into muffin cups, filling them almost full. Bake until muffins have risen slightly and are golden brown, 25-30 minutes. Remove from cups.
Yield: 12 muffins

Recipe notes: If sunflower seeds are raw, spread them out in a pie plate and toast them in a 375 F oven, stirring once, until one shade darker, about 5 minutes.

🍎🍎🍎🍎🍎

Per serving: 162 Calories; 6.9g Fat (satfat 0.7g); 4g Protein; 23g Carbohydrate; 15mg Cholesterol; 180mg Sodium

Sweet Muffins

2	egg whites or 2 tablespoons tofu
1	cup skim milk
1/4	cup margarine
2	cups unbleached flour
1/4	cup honey
3	teaspoons baking powder
1	teaspoon salt

Beat eggs; stir in milk and oil. Mix in remaining ingredients just until flour is moistened. Batter should be lumpy. Fill muffin tins 2/3 full. Bake 20-25 minutes or until golden brown, at 400°. Immediately remove from pan.
Yield: 12 muffins

Variations on a Theme
APPLE MUFFINS: Stir in 1 cup grated apple with the oil and add 1/2-teaspoon cinnamon with the flour. Sprinkle with Nut-Crunch Topping: mix 1/3-cup fructose, 1/3-cup nuts, chopped and 1/2 teaspoon cinnamon.
WHOLE WHEAT MUFFINS: decrease flour to 1 cup and baking powder to 2 teaspoons; add 1 cup whole wheat flour.
SURPRISE MUFFINS: fill muffin tins half full of batter; drop 1 teaspoon jelly or peanut butter in center and add rest of batter to 2/3 full.

🍎🍎🍎🍎🍎

Per serving: 117 Calories; less than one gram Fat (satfat 0.1g); 3g Protein; 25g Carbohydrate; 0mg Cholesterol; 289mg Sodium

Poppy Seed Muffins

3	cups unbleached flour
2	tablespoons poppy seeds
1 1/2	teaspoons baking powder
1 1/2	teaspoons salt
3	flax seed eggs or 2 egg whites + 1 egg
1 1/2	cups apple juice, frozen concentrate
1/2	cup canola oil
1/2	cup yogurt
1 1/2	teaspoons vanilla extract
1 1/2	teaspoons almond extract

In a large bowl, combine flour, sugar, poppy seeds, baking powder and salt. In another bowl, beat eggs, milk, oil and extracts; stir into dry ingredients just until moistened. Fill greased or paper-lined muffin cups two-thirds full. Bake at 350 for 20-25 minutes or until muffins test done. Cool in pan 10 minutes before removing to a wire rack.
Yield: 24 muffins

Per serving: 102 Calories; 0.5g Fat (satfat 0.1g); 1.8g Protein; 22.4g Carbohydrate; 0 mg Cholesterol; 161mg Sodium

Pumpkin Chip Muffins

1	eggs
3	egg whites *or* 2 flax seed eggs
1 1/4	cups natural sugar or fructose
16	ounces pumpkin, canned
3/4	cup apple juice, frozen concentrate
3/4	cup applesauce, unsweetened
3	cups all-purpose flour
2	teaspoons baking soda
2	tablespoons baking powder
1	teaspoon cinnamon
1	teaspoon salt
2	cups semisweet chocolate chips

In a large mixing bowl, beat eggs, sugar, pumpkin and oil until smooth. Combine flour, baking soda, baking powder, cinnamon and salt; add to pumpkin mixture and mix well. Fold in chocolate chips. Fill greased or paper lined muffin cups three-fourths full. Bake at 400° for 16-20 minutes or until muffins test done. Cool in pan 10 minutes before removing to a wire rack.
Yield: 24 muffins

Per serving: 184 Calories; 5g Fat (satfat 2.6); 3g Protein; 35g Carbohydrate; 8mg Cholesterol; 300mg Sodium

Peachy Almond Muffins

1 1/2	cups all-purpose flour
3/4	cup fructose or natural sugar
3/4	teaspoon salt
1/2	teaspoon baking soda
3	egg whites or 2 flax seed eggs
1/4	cup softened margarine or soy margarine
1/4	cup frozen apple juice concentrate
1/2	teaspoon vanilla extract
1/8	teaspoon almond extract
1 1/4	cups fresh peaches, chopped and peeled
1 1/4	cups almonds,chopped

In a large bowl, combine flour, sugar, salt and baking soda. In another bowl, beat eggs, margarine, apple juice and extracts; stir into dry ingredients just until moistened. Fold in peaches and almonds. Fill greased or paper-lined muffin cups three-fourths full. Bake at 375 for 20-25 minutes or until muffins test done. Cool in pan for 10 minutes before removing to a wire rack. *Yield: 12 muffins*
Variation on a Theme
A 16-oz. can of peaches, drained and chopped can be substituted for the fresh peaches.

🍎🍎🍎🍎🍎

Per serving: 143 Calories; 3g Fat (satfat 0.6g); 3g Protein; 26g Carbohydrate; 0mg Cholesterol; 236mg Sodium

Pancakes

1 1/2	cups unbleached flour
1	tablespoon baking powder
2	tablespoons honey
1/2	teaspoon salt
1	egg or 2 tablespoons tofu
1 1/4	cups skim milk
1/2	cup applesauce *or* canola oil

Stir flour, baking powder, sugar, and salt together in a wide mouth jar, a quart measuring pitcher, or a medium bowl, mixing thoroughly. Beat in egg and oil. The batter will be a little lumpy. Preheat griddle. Pour batter onto griddle sprayed lightly with vegetable spray. Bake until the pancake is full of bubbles, then it is ready to flip over. Cook other side until golden brown, then remove with spatula. For variety try adding grated apples, blueberries, chopped nuts, cinnamon, or just anything you can conjure up. Yield: 12 pancakes

🍎🍎🍎🍎🍎

Per serving: 102 Calories; 1.7g Fat (satfat 0.4g); 3g Protein; 16g Carbohydrate; 16mg Cholesterol; 198mg Sodium

Zucchini Carrot Muffins

2	cups carrots, shredded
1	cup zucchini, shredded
1	cup apple, peeled and chopped
3/4	cup coconut, flaked
1/2	cup almonds, chopped
2	teaspoons orange peel, grated
2	cups unbleached flour
1	cup fructose or natural sugar
1	tablespoon cinnamon
2	tablespoons baking soda
1/2	teaspoon salt
1	egg + 3 egg whites, lightly beaten
3/4	cup applesauce, unsweetened
1	teaspoon vanilla extract

Gently toss together carrot, zucchini, apple, coconut, almonds and orange peel; set aside. In a large bowl, combine flour, sugar, cinnamon, baking soda and salt. Combine eggs, oil and vanilla; stir into dry ingredients just until moistened (batter will be thick). Fold in carrot mixture. Fill greased or paper-lined muffin cups two-thirds full. Bake at 375° for 20-22 minutes or until muffins test done. Cool in pan 10 minutes before removing to a wire rack.
Yield: 18 muffins

Per serving: 119 Calories; 2g Fat (satfat 0.7g); 3g Protein; 24g Carbohydrate; 10mg Cholesterol; 497mg Sodium

Herbed Oatmeal Pan Bread

Breads

1 1/2	cups boiling water
1	cup oats, rolled (raw)
2	packages active dry yeast
1/2	cup warm water, 110° to 115°
1/4	cup fructose or natural sugar
3	tablespoons margarine, softened
2	teaspoons salt
1	egg, lightly beaten
4	cups all-purpose flour
	TOPPING
1/4	cup margarine, melted & divided
2	tablespoons Parmesan cheese, grated
1	teaspoon dried basil
1/2	teaspoon dried oregano
1/2	teaspoon garlic powder

In a small bowl, combine boiling water and oats; cool to 110-115 degrees. In a mixing bowl, dissolve yeast in warm water. Add sugar, butter, salt, egg, oat mixture and 2 cups of flour; beat until smooth. Add enough remaining flour to form soft dough. Turn onto a floured board; knead until smooth and elastic, about 6-8 minutes. Place in a greased bowl, turning once to grease top. Cover and let rise in a warm place until doubled, about 30 minutes.

Punch dough down and press evenly into a greased 13-in. x 9-in. x 2-in. baking pan. With a very sharp knife, cut diagonal lines 1-1/2 in. apart completely through dough. Repeat in opposite direction, creating a diamond pattern. Cover and let rise in a warm place until doubled, about 1 hour.

Redefine pattern by gently poking along cut lines with knife tip. Brush with 2 tablespoons melted butter. Bake at 375 for 15 minutes. Meanwhile, combine Parmesan cheese, basil, oregano and garlic powder. Brush bread with remaining butter; sprinkle with cheese mixture. Bake for 5 minutes. Loosely cover with foil and bake 5 minutes longer. Serve warm.
Yield: 16 slices

🍎🍎🍎🍎🍎

Per serving: 185 Calories; 4g Fat (satfat 1.0g); 5g Protein; 30g Carbohydrate; 12mg Cholesterol; 328mg Sodium

Icebox Butterhorns

1	package active dry yeast
2	tablespoons warm water 110° to 115°
2	cups skim milk 110-115°
1/3	cup fructose or natural sugar
1	egg or 2 tablespoons tofu
1	teaspoon salt
6	cups all-purpose flour
3/4	cup margarine, melted
	additional melted margarine

In a large mixing bowl, dissolve yeast in water. Add milk, sugar, egg, salt and 3 cups flour; beat until smooth. Fold in margarine and remaining flour (dough will be slightly sticky). Do not knead. Place in a greased bowl. Cover and refrigerate overnight. Punch dough down and divide in half.

On a floured surface, roll each half into a 12-in. circle. Cut each circle into 12 pie-shaped wedges. Beginning at the wide end, roll up each wedge. Place rolls point side down, 2 in. apart on greased baking sheets. Cover and let rise in a warm place until doubled, about 1 hour. Bake at 350° for 15-20 minutes or until golden brown. Immediately brush tops with melted butter.
Yield: 24 rolls

🍎🍎🍎🍎🍎

Per serving: 168 Calories; 4g Fat (satfat 0.9g); 4g Protein; 27g Carbohydrate; 8mg Cholesterol; 153mg Sodium

Granny's Whole Wheat Bread

3/4	cup milk, scalded
2	tablespoons honey
4	teaspoons salt
1/3	cup molasses
2	tablespoons yeast
1	teaspoon fructose or natural sugar
2	cups warm water
4 1/2	cups whole wheat flour
2 1/2	cups flour

Scald 3/4-cup milk; add honey, salt and molasses. Soften 2 tablespoons yeast in 1 1/2 cups warm water with a teaspoon of sugar added. Add flour and let rise twice and once more in pan not quite double in bulk. Bake at 375 degrees for 15 minutes then 325 for 30 minutes.
Yield: 24 slices

🍎🍎🍎🍎🍎

Per serving: 149 Calories; 1g Fat (satfat 0.3g); 5g Protein; 32g Carbohydrate; 1mg Cholesterol; 363mg Sodium

Pumpkin Bread

2	cups pumpkin, canned
1/2	cup canola oil
2	egg whites *or* 2 tablespoons tofu
1/3	cup plain lowfat yogurt
3 1/2	cups unbleached flour
2/3	cup apple juice, frozen concentrate
1/2	cup brown sugar
1/2	teaspoon salt
1	teaspoon cinnamon
1/2	teaspoon ginger
1/2	teaspoon allspice
1/2	teaspoon nutmeg
2 1/2	teaspoons baking soda

Mix together pumpkin, oil, egg and yogurt. Add remaining ingredients and mix well. Pour into 3 well greased bread pans. Bake one hour at 350°F or until toothpick comes out clean. If you want can put a thin glaze of powdered sugar, butter, milk and almond flavoring on the warm bread.
Yield: 3 loaves

🍎🍎🍎🍎🍎🍎

Per serving: 55 Calories; 0.2g Fat (satfat 0.1); 1.3g Protein; 12.1g Carbohydrate; 0mg Cholesterol; 79mg Sodium

Whole Wheat Pizza Crust

1	package active dry yeast
1/2	cup warm water
1 1/2	cups whole wheat flour
1/4	teaspoon salt
1	tablespoon canola oil

Stir yeast into water in a bowl. Mix in flour, salt, and oil. Knead mixture on a lightly floured surface until it forms a smooth ball. Place in a greased bowl, turn once to grease surface. Cover and let rise in a warm place about 15 minutes. Grease deep-dish pizza pan with solid shortening. Press dough into bottom and around in pan. Bake at 450 for 10 minutes, then remove and add pizza sauce (3/4 cup) over dough. Top with cheese and any other desired ingredients. Return to oven for 10-15 minutes or until cheese is melted. *Yield: 1 pizza crust*

🍎🍎🍎🍎🍎🍎

Per serving: 96 Calories; 2g Fat (satfat 0.2g); 4g Protein; 17g Carbohydrate; 0mg Cholesterol; 69mg Sodium

Oatmeal Wheat Bread

1 3/4	cups boiling water
1	cup quick-cooking oats
1/2	cup molasses
1/4	cup canola oil
1/4	cup orange juice
1 1/2	teaspoons salt
2	packages active dry yeast
1/2	cup warm water 110° to 115°
2 1/2	cups whole wheat flour
3	cups all-purpose flour
	melted margarine

In a large mixing bowl, combine boiling water, oats, molasses, shortening, orange juice and salt; let stand until warm (110-115 degrees). In a small bowl, dissolve yeast in warm water; add to oat mixture. Add whole-wheat flour and beat until smooth. Add enough all-purpose flour to form soft dough. Turn onto a floured board; knead until smooth and elastic, about 6-8 minutes. Place in a greased bowl, turning once to grease top. Cover and let rise in a warm place until doubled, about 1 hour. Punch dough down. Shape into two loaves; place in greased 8-in. x 4-in. x 2-in. loaf pans. Cover and let rise until doubled, about 45 minutes. Bake at 350° for 40 minutes. Remove from pans; brush with margarine. Cool on wire racks.
Yield: 2 loaves or about 32 slices

Per serving: 116 Calories; 2g Fat (satfat 0.2g); 3g Protein; 21g Carbohydrate; 0mg Cholesterol; 104mg Sodium

Whole Wheat Cinnamon Rolls

2	cakes yeast
2	cups warm water
1/4	cup honey
2	eggs or 2 flax seed eggs, well beaten
1/3	cup margarine or soy margarine
2	teaspoons salt
1	teaspoon cardamom, optional
2/3	cup powdered milk
4 1/2	cups whole wheat flour
1	cup powdered sugar
1	teaspoon maple flavoring

Dissolve yeast in 1/2-cup warm water and 1/2 cup sugar. Add 2 well-beaten eggs, 1-1/2 cups warm water, butter, salt cardamom, 2/3 cup powdered milk and wheat flour that was stirred but not sifted. Make soft dough, let rise 2-3 times. Roll out and sprinkle with a cinnamon and sugar mixture. Roll up, as for jellyroll. Cut into slices, let rise until light. Fry at 400 degrees in deep fat until brown, drain and dip into glaze and set on rack to drain. Glaze is made from 1 cup of powdered sugar, 1-teaspoon maple flavoring and hot water.
Yield: 24 rolls

🍎🍎🍎🍎🍎🍎

Per serving: 148 Calories; 3g Fat (satfat 1.1g); 5g Protein; 26g Carbohydrate; 19mg Cholesterol; 220mg Sodium

French Bread

1	tablespoon dry yeast
1 1/2	cups warm water
1	teaspoon salt
1	tablespoon margarine
4 1/2	cups unbleached flour
2	teaspoons cornmeal

In a large mixing bowl, dissolve yeast in warm water. Add salt, butter, and 2 cups flour. Beat with spoon until thoroughly mixed. Gradually add remaining flour until dough is easy to handle. Kneed on a lightly floured board for five to ten minutes or until dough is elastic and not sticky. Place in a greased bowl with plastic wrap. Let rise in a warm place until double in size. 1-1 1/2 hours. Punch down and place on a lightly floured surface. Divide into two equal pieces. Shape each piece into a long narrow loaf, about 14" long and 1 1/2 inches in diameter. Lightly grease inside of French Bread pans (you can use a cookie sheet, but they will not be as uniform) Sprinkle 1 teaspoon cornmeal in each section. Shake pan to distribute evenly. Place loaves in pan. With sharp knife make three or four diagonal 1/4" deep slashes on the top of each loaf. Do not cover. Let rise in a warm place until double in size, about 45 minutes. Bake in preheated oven 375 for 25 to 30 minutes. Remove from pans at once. Serve hot or cold.

Yield: 18 slices

🍎🍎🍎🍎🍎🍎

Per serving: 121 Calories; 1g Fat (satfat 0.1g); 4g Protein; 24g Carbohydrate; 0mg Cholesterol; 125mg Sodium

Quickie Hamburger Buns

3 1/2	cups warm water
1/2	cup oil
1/2	cup honey
6	tablespoons yeast
1	tablespoon salt
2	eggs, whites + 1 egg
8	cups whole wheat flour
2 1/2	cups unbleached flour

Mix water, oil, sugar and yeast and set aside for 15 minutes. Then add salt, eggs and flour, mixing thoroughly.

Shape immediately into rolls, cinnamon rolls, or hamburger buns. To make hamburger buns shape dough into size and shape of a hamburger patty. Twelve hamburger buns fit on a cookie sheet. Let rise about 10 minutes and bake 10 minutes at 425 degrees. *Yield: 8 dozen rolls or 2 dozen hamburger buns.*

Variation on a Theme
Try different types of flour, Like my seven-grain mix.

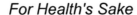

Per serving: 64 Calories; 1.4g Fat (satfat 0.2g); 2g Protein; 11g Carbohydrate; 4mg Cholesterol; 70mg Sodium

Zola's Bread

3	cups warm water
4	tablespoons honey
4	tablespoons dry yeast
4	cups wheat flour
2	cups skim milk *or* soy milk
2	tablespoons salt
1/3	cup canola oil
10	cups flour
4	tablespoons honey

Measure into bowl, mix and let stand until dissolved: warm water, honey, and yeast. Add 4 cups wheat flour and stir well. Beat until smooth, cover and let rise in warm place until spongy. , for about 30 minutes or more. Scald milk. Add honey, salt, and oil. Let cool to room temperature, then add to sponge and mix well. When sponge is light stir in. Add 8 cups flour, mix well. Knead for 5 to 10 minutes incorporating in no more than 2 cups flour. (It will be slightly sticky) Cover and let rise until doubled, punch down and let rise again. Let rise only 45 minutes the second time. Shape into loaves, and rise again. Bake 400° for 25-30 minutes. Cool on wire rack.
Yields: 4-5 loaves.

Per serving: 119 Calories; 2g Fat (satfat 0.1g); 4g Protein; 23g Carbohydrate; 0mg Cholesterol; 205mg Sodium

Fruits and Veggies

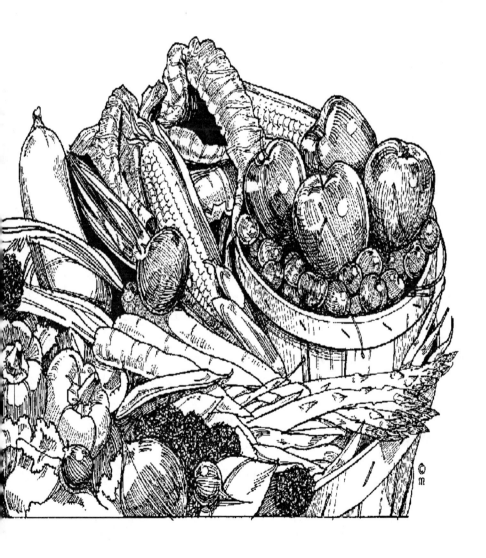

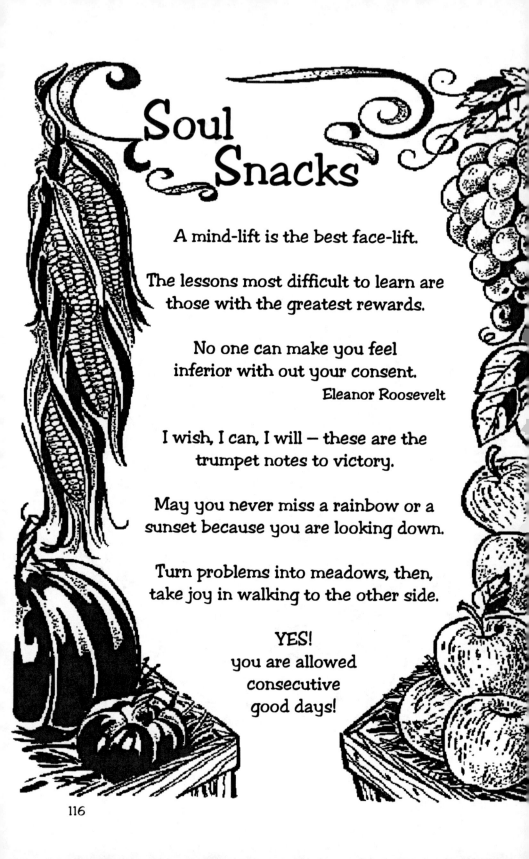

Soul
Snacks

A mind-lift is the best face-lift.

The lessons most difficult to learn are
those with the greatest rewards.

No one can make you feel
inferior with out your consent.

Eleanor Roosevelt

I wish, I can, I will — these are the
trumpet notes to victory.

May you never miss a rainbow or a
sunset because you are looking down.

Turn problems into meadows, then,
take joy in walking to the other side.

YES!
you are allowed
consecutive
good days!

Apple Gratin

2	pounds Granny Smith apple, peeled and sliced
1/2	cup raisins
1/2	teaspoon cinnamon
1/4	cup lemon juice
1/2	cup brown sugar, packed
1/2	cup unbleached flour
	dash salt
1/4	cup margarine
2/3	cup sharp cheddar cheese, lowfat

In a well-buttered 1-quart casserole arrange apple slices. Sprinkle with raisins, cinnamon, and lemon juice (for sweeter apples use less lemon juice). Cut together with a fork: brown sugar, flour, salt, margarine and cheese. Sprinkle over the apples. Bake at 350° for 30 minutes or until apples are tender.
Yield: 8 servings

🍎🍎🍎🍎🍎

Per serving: 203 Calories; 4g Fat (satfat 1.2); 4g Protein; 36g Carbohydrate; 2mg Cholesterol; 115mg Sodium

Orange Appetizer

2	large oranges, diced
4	tablespoons pineapple chunks in juice

Peel, dice, and remove seeds from oranges. Put into each glass 1/2 diced orange and 2 tablespoons chunk pineapple. Stir and set in refrigerator until time to serve.

Yield: 4 servings

Variations on a Theme

Add sliced strawberries or seeded purple grapes. Add 1-tablespoon lime juice and slices of papaya, quava, or diced mango or kumquat. Instead of pineapple use sliced fresh apricots, peaches, plums, or California persimmons; diced cantaloupe or Persian melon; seeded or seedless grapes; seeded cherries and/or white cherries; grapefruit sections or wedges or unpeeled yellow pear or plum.

🍎🍎🍎🍎🍎

Per serving: 35 Calories; less than one gram Fat (satfat 0g); 1g Protein; 13g Carbohydrate; 0mg Cholesterol; 1mg Sodium

Pineapple Boats
These pineapple boats look great on a buffet table

1	large fresh pineapple
4	large carrots, grated
3	stalks celery, diced
1/2	cup pecans, chopped
1/2	cup seedless raisins

Sauce

2/3	cup lowfat cottage cheese *or* soy yogurt
2	tablespoons apple cider vinegar
1/3	cup pineapple juice
2	tablespoons honey
3	tablespoons canola oil
1	teaspoon lemon juice

Cut pineapple in half lengthwise and scoop out the insides, then cut into cubes. Grate carrots, dice celery and chop nuts. Place pineapple, carrots, celery, nuts and raisin in a large bowl. Prepare sauce by putting all ingredients in blender and mix on high speed until creamy. Pour sauce over fruit and mix until everything is coated and mixed well. Then take mix and pile it inside the empty pineapple shells. This makes quite a lot and it will not all fit back in the pineapple shells, so just save it in the fridge or place in desert bowls and sprinkle with fresh grated coconut.
Yield: 10 servings

🍎🍎🍎🍎🍎

Per serving: 158 Calories; 7g Fat (satfat 0.6g); 3g Protein; 24g Carbohydrate; 1mg Cholesterol; 81mg Sodium

Yogurt Fruit Cup

1	slice cantaloupe, diced
1/3	cup blueberries
2	wedges apple, diced
8	seedless green grapes, halved
3	tablespoons wheat germ
2/3	cup plain nonfat yogurt

Combine all ingredients into a cereal bowl and mix well. Yield: 1 serving

🍎🍎🍎🍎🍎

Per serving: 448 Calories; 4g Fat (satfat 0.7); 16g Protein; 96g Carbohydrate; 3mg Cholesterol; 146mg Sodium

Baby Carrots with Curry Sauce

1	pound baby carrots
3	tablespoons light mayonnaise *or* soy mayonnaise
3	tablespoons light sour cream *or* soy sour cream
1	teaspoon curry powder
1	teaspoon skim milk *or* soy milk
1	teaspoon fresh lemon juice
1	teaspoon honey

Steam carrots, covered, 7 minutes or until crisp-tender; drain.

Combine mayonnaise, sour cream, curry powder, milk, lemon juice and honey
in a saucepan; place over medium-low heat until hot, stirring occasionally. Just
before serving pour sauce over carrots.
Yield: 4 servings

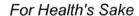

Per serving: 66 Calories; 1g Fat (satfat 0.4); 1g Protein; 13g Carbohydrate;
6mg Cholesterol; 100mg Sodium

Bean Sprout Casserole

2	cups bean sprouts
3	tablespoons green pepper, chopped
1	cup corn, frozen
2	cups Basic White Sauce (page 157)
	salt and pepper
	buttered crumbs

Make Basic White Sauce. Toss together bean sprouts, green pepper, corn and
white sauce. Place in greased casserole. Top with crumbs. Bake at 350° for
25 minutes.
Yield: 4 servings

Per serving: 77 Calories; 2g Fat (satfat 0.3); 3g Protein; 13g Carbohydrate;
0mg Cholesterol; 12mg Sodium

Brussel Sprouts With Yogurt

2 1/2	pounds brussel sprouts
1	medium tomato, chopped
2	tablespoons fresh chives, chopped
1/2	teaspoon nutmeg
	salt and pepper
1	cup plain lowfat yogurt or soy yogurt
1/4	cup Kraft Free® nonfat grated topping *or* soy Parmesan cheese
1/4	cup sliced almonds

Drop the brussel sprouts into boiling salted water, and cook for about 10 minutes, or until they are tender. Remove the sprouts from the heat and drain thoroughly. Place the sprouts in a buttered ovenproof casserole; cover them with the tomato and chives. Sprinkle the vegetables with nutmeg and season them with salt and pepper. Pour the yogurt over them. Sprinkle the top with the grated cheese and toasted almonds, bake for 15 minutes in an oven, preheated to 350° until the top is nicely browned. Serve hot.
Yield: 4 servings

🍎🍎🍎🍎🍎🍎

Per serving: 207 Calories; 7g Fat (satfat 1.3g); 14g Protein; 30g Carbohydrate; 3mg Cholesterol; 107mg Sodium

Chinese Style Vegetable Medley

1	small head of cabbage
1	tablespoon fat-free chicken broth or vegetarian broth
1	cup celery thinly sliced
1	medium green pepper cut diagonal
2/3	cup onion, chopped
1/2	teaspoon salt
1/8	teaspoon pepper

Prepare 3 cups finely shredded cabbage. Heat broth in medium skillet. Add vegetables and stir. Cover; steam 5 minutes or until crisp-tender, stirring several times. Add salt and pepper. If desired, stir in 1-tablespoon soy sauce.
Yield: 4 servings

🍎🍎🍎🍎🍎🍎

Per serving: 36 Calories; less than one gram Fat (satfat 0g); 2g Protein; 8g Carbohydrate; 0mg Cholesterol; 413mg Sodium

Copper Pennies

2	pounds sliced carrot
2	medium onions cut into rings
1	green pepper, sliced in strips
1	can tomato soup
3	tablespoons olive oil
1/3	cup orange juice frozen concentrate, thawed
1/2	cup honey
1	teaspoon Worcestershire sauce
1	teaspoon mustard
1/2	teaspoon salt

Cook carrots in salted water till tender. Drain. Combine with onion and green pepper in large bowl. Stir together remaining ingredients and pour over vegetables. Cover and marinate in refrigerator overnight. Drain, save marinade. Serve in lettuce lined bowl. Return left over vegetables to marinade and refrigerate. Marinade may be used as salad dressing.
Yield: 6 servings

🍎🍎🍎🍎🍎

Per serving: 250 Calories; 7g Fat (satfat 1.0g); 3g Protein; 47g Carbohydrate; 0mg Cholesterol; 574mg Sodium

Creamed Peas and Potatoes

4	medium red potatoes, cubed
10	ounces frozen peas
2	tablespoons margarine or soy margarine
2	tablespoons unbleached flour
1/2	teaspoon salt
1/4	teaspoon white pepper
1 1/2	cups skim milk or soy milk
1	tablespoon Herbes de Provence or Italian Seasoning
1	dash garlic powder

Place potatoes in a saucepan; cover with water and cook until tender. Cook peas according to package directions, adding the sugar. Meanwhile, melt butter in a saucepan; add flour, salt and pepper to form a paste. Gradually stir in milk. Bring to a boil; boil for 1 minute. Add Herbes de Provence; cook until thickened and bubbly. Drain potatoes and peas; place in a serving bowl. Pour sauce over vegetables and stir till evenly coated. Serve immediately.
Yield: 6 servings

🍎🍎🍎🍎🍎

Per serving: 153 Calories; 4g Fat (satfat 0.8g); 6g Protein; 23g Carbohydrate; 1mg Cholesterol; 311mg Sodium

Curried Green Beans and Potatoes

1	pound red potatoes or (3 cups) halved lengthwise and sliced
2 1/2	cups frozen green beans
1 1/2	teaspoons curry powder
1/2	teaspoon salt
1/2	teaspoon cumin seed, crushed
1/4	teaspoon ginger
1/8	teaspoon pepper
1	cup plain nonfat yogurt or soy yogurt
1	clove garlic, minced
1	tablespoon dry-roasted peanuts, chopped

Place potato slices in a medium saucepan; cover with water, and bring to a boil over medium-high heat. Cover and cook 5 minutes. Add green beans, and cook, uncovered, 8 minutes or until the vegetables are tender. Drain and set aside.

Combine curry powder and next 4 ingredients in a large nonstick skillet; cook over low heat 5 minutes. Stir in yogurt and garlic; cook just until mixture is warm. (Do not overcook or yogurt will separate.)
Combine potato mixture and yogurt mixture in a large bowl; toss gently. Sprinkle with peanuts.
Yield: 6 servings

🍎🍎🍎🍎🍎

Per serving: 98 Calories; 2g Fat (satfat 0.5g); 5g Protein; 18g Carbohydrate; 2mg Cholesterol; 222mg Sodium

Toasty Cauliflower and Broccoli

4	cups fresh or frozen cauliflower florets
4	cups fresh or frozen broccoli florets
2	cloves garlic, chopped
2	teaspoons olive oil
1/4	teaspoon salt
	Vegetable cooking spray

Combine cauliflower florets, broccoli florets, and garlic in a large bowl. Add olive oil and salt, and toss well to coat. Arrange the mixture in a single layer in a 13 x 9-inch baking dish coated with cooking spray. Bake at 400° degrees for 30 minutes or until tender and lightly browned, stirring every 5 minutes.
Yield: 4 servings

🍎🍎🍎🍎🍎

Per serving: 92 Calories; 3g Fat (satfat 0.4g); 7g Protein; 14g Carbohydrate; 0mg Cholesterol; 190mg Sodium

Dilly Carrots

1	pound baby carrots
1/2	small onion, halved
2	cloves garlic
2	teaspoons salt
1/8	teaspoon cayenne pepper
1	tablespoon fresh dill weed
1	tablespoon dill seed
1 1/4	cups vinegar
1 1/4	cups water

Cut carrots into lengthwise slices that will fit a pint-size jar. Pack into two pint-sized jars. In each jar, also place a piece of onion, a garlic clove, 1 teaspoons of salt, 1/2 tablespoon of dill weed, 1/2-tablespoon dill seed, and a pinch of cayenne pepper. Bring vinegar and water to a boil. Pour over carrots. Store in refrigerator, or process jars according to manufacturers' instructions. Wait until chilled to serve.
Yield: 2 pints or 6 -8 servings

Variation on a Theme
To make dilly green beans, substitute whole fresh green beans, washed, trimmed, and blanched, for carrots

🍎🍎🍎🍎🍎

Per serving: 43 Calories; 1g Fat (satfat 0.1g); 1g Protein; 11g Carbohydrate; 0mg Cholesterol; 785mg Sodium

Green Beans With Garlic

1 1/2	pounds green beans, trimmed & cut	
2	tablespoons olive oil	
6	cloves garlic	crushed
3	cups fresh bread crumbs	
	salt and pepper	

Heat the olive oil in a large skillet and, when hot, throw in the garlic cloves. When the garlic begins to turn transparent, add the green beans and stir with a wooden spoon. Keep the oil very hot. When beans start to turn dark green, add the bread crumbs and stir briskly so that they do not burn or stick to the bottom of the pan. Turn the mixture immediately onto a warmed platter. Add salt and pepper to taste, and serve at once. *Yield: 8 servings*

🍎🍎🍎🍎🍎

Per serving: 22 Calories; 6g Fat (satfat 1.1g); 6g Protein; 36g Carbohydrate; 0mg Cholesterol; 288mg Sodium

Garden Stir Fry

1	teaspoon canola oil
1	cup sliced onion, separated into rings
1	cup red bell pepper, sliced into rings
2	cloves garlic minced
1 3/4	cups yellow squash, sliced
1 3/4	cups zucchini, sliced
1	cup plum tomatoes, chopped
1	tablespoon basil
1/2	teaspoon lemon pepper
1/4	teaspoon salt
2	tablespoons Parmesan cheese or soy Parmesan cheese

Heat oil in a large nonstick skillet over medium-high heat. Add onion, bell pepper, and garlic; stir-fry 2 minutes. Add squash and zucchini; stir-fry 3 minutes or until vegetables are crisp-tender. Add tomato and next 3 ingredients; cook 1 minute or until thoroughly heated. Remove from heat; sprinkle with cheese. Serve immediately.
Yield: 5 servings

🍎🍎🍎🍎🍎

Per serving: 61 Calories; 2g Fat (satfat 0.5g); 3g Protein; 10g Carbohydrate; 2mg Cholesterol; 185mg Sodium

Garlicky Smashed Potatoes and Carrots

6	cups potato, cubed
1/2	cup carrot, thinly sliced
4	cloves garlic, peeled
3/4	cup buttermilk *or* soy milk + lemon juice
1/2	teaspoon salt
1/4	teaspoon pepper
1	Dash ground nutmeg

Combine first 3 ingredients in a saucepan; add water to cover, and bring to a boil. Cover, reduce heat, and simmer 15 minutes or until very tender; drain well.

Combine potato mixture, buttermilk, and remaining ingredients in a bowl; beat at medium speed of electric mixer 2 minutes or until smooth.
Yield: 6 servings

Personal Note: I almost always leave the skins on my potatoes, unless they are tough. It gives added fiber and vitamins.

🍎🍎🍎🍎🍎

Per serving: 68 Calories; less than one gram Fat (satfat 0.2g); 2g Protein; 14g Carbohydrate; 1mg Cholesterol; 220mg Sodium

Marinated Vegetables

1	can fat-free chicken broth or vegetarian broth
1/4	cup vinegar
1	tablespoon olive oil
1	package Italian salad dressing mix
2	cups zucchini, thinly sliced
1	cup broccoli flowerets
1	cup cauliflower, sliced
1	cup mushrooms, sliced
1	cup cherry tomatoes cut in half
1	cup onion slices
2	cups carrot slices

In small saucepan, boil broth and carrots 3 minutes. Cool. Mix dressing of vinegar, oil and broth and blend well. Combine vegetables in shallow dish, pour in marinate, cover and chill 6 hours or more. Stir occasionally.
Yield: 10 servings

🍎🍎🍎🍎🍎

Per serving: 57 Calories; 2g Fat (satfat 0.3g); 3g Protein; 8g Carbohydrate; 0mg Cholesterol; 271mg Sodium

Minted Peas

2	cups frozen peas
4	springs fresh mint leaves
1/2	cup water

Place frozen peas and mint leaves into 1/2 cup boiling water. Bring to a second boil. Reduce heat; cover and cook gently about 10 minutes or until tender. Do not overcook. Drain and remove mint leaves before serving. Serve hot or cold.
Yield: 4 servings.

Personal Note: If you can't find fresh mint leaves then do the next best thing hang a herbal tea bag in with your vegetables while they cook you will achieve comparable results. You might also try different herbal teas with your vegetables to get different taste sensations.

🍎🍎🍎🍎🍎

Per serving: 56 Calories; less than one gram Fat (satfat 0); 4g Protein; 10g Carbohydrate; 0mg Cholesterol; 82mg Sodium

New Potatoes with Chopped Mushrooms

1 1/4	pounds new potatoes, washed
2	tablespoons canola or corn oil
1	scallion, chopped
1 1/2	cups mushrooms finely chopped
2	tablespoons flour
1 1/2	cups fat-free chicken broth or vegetarian broth
1	bay leaf
2	teaspoons parsley, finely chopped

Boil the potatoes in salted water until tender - about 15 minutes. Drain and set them aside. Heat the oil in a heavy saucepan. Sauté the scallion in the oil for 2 to 3 minutes. Add the flour and stir until smoothly mixed. Gradually add the stock, stirring all the time until smooth. Add the bay leaf and bring the mixture to a boil, then reduce the heat and simmer, uncovered for 8 minutes. Add the cooked potatoes to the sauce and stirring occasionally heat through over low heat. Taste and adjust the seasoning. Sprinkle with the parsley or mint and serve.
Yield: 4 servings

🍎🍎🍎🍎🍎

Per serving: 151 Calories; 4g Fat (satfat 0.8g); 8g Protein; 25g Carbohydrate; 0mg Cholesterol; 255mg Sodium

Onion-Roasted Potatoes

2	pounds red potatoes, sliced 1/2" thick
1	envelope onion soup mix
	Butter flavored vegetable spray

Place potatoes in large plastic bag and spray with vegetable spray until potatoes are well coated. Add onion soup mix and shake until evenly coated. Place 3 tablespoons of water in bottom of pan. Empty bag onto a 13x9-in.-baking pan sprayed with vegetable spray. Cover and bake at 350° for 35 minutes, stirring occasionally. Uncover, lightly spray potatoes with vegetable spray and bake another 10-15 minutes or until potatoes are tender.
Yield: 6 servings

🍎🍎🍎🍎🍎

Per serving: 109 Calories; less than one gram Fat (satfat 0.1g); 3g Protein; 24g Carbohydrate; 0mg Cholesterol; 589mg Sodium

Orange Candied Sweet Potatoes

6	medium sweet potato cooked and peeled
1	small orange, peeled & thinly sliced
1/3	cup brown sugar, packed
1	teaspoon salt
1	tablespoon orange peel, grated
4	tablespoons margarine *or* soy margarine, sliced

Cut sweet potatoes in 1/2" slices. Place half the slice in greased 2-quart casserole. Top with orange slices, then half the sugar, salt and orange peel. Dot with half the butter. Add remaining sweet potatoes. Top with remaining sugar, salt, orange peels and butter. Bake uncovered in 375° oven for 30 minutes or until glazed.

Yield: 6 servings

🍎🍎🍎🍎🍎🍎

Per serving: 183 Calories; 5g Fat (satfat 1.1g); 2g Protein; 33g Carbohydrate; 0mg Cholesterol; 437mg Sodium

Parmesan Cauliflower

1	large head cauliflower
3	tablespoons toasted breadcrumbs
2	tablespoons Parmesan cheese *or* soy Parmesan cheese
	Butter flavored vegetable spray
	Paprika

Separate cauliflower into flowerets. Cook in small amount of boiling salted water until tender, about 10 minutes. Drain. Coat cooked cauliflower with butter flavored vegetable spray; toss with breadcrumbs. Sprinkle cheese over top. Garnish with paprika.

Yield: 4 servings

🍎🍎🍎🍎🍎🍎

Per serving: 34 Calories; 1g Fat (satfat 0.6g); 2g Protein; 4g Carbohydrate; 2mg Cholesterol; 85mg Sodium

Ranch Hand Beans

1	pound dried pinto beans
6	cups water
1	teaspoon salt
2	cups onion chopped
1	clove garlic, minced
12	ounces Morningstar Farms® Harvest Burgers Recipe Crumbles *or* 1 pound extra lean ground beef
1	12 oz-can diced tomatoes
1	tablespoon chili powder
1	green pepper, diced
1	teaspoon salt
1/2	teaspoon cumin
1/2	teaspoon marjoram

Wash beans. Combine beans and water in Dutch Oven. Bring to a boil; boil 2 minutes. Remove from heat; cover and let stand 1 hour (or soak overnight). Add 1-teaspoon salt, onion, garlic, green peppers, and crumbles or ground beef. Bring to a boil. Reduce heat, cover and let simmer about 2 hours or until beans are tender. Drain beans, reserving 1-cup liquid. Add tomatoes, chili powder, 1-teaspoon salt, cumin and marjoram. Stir in reserved liquid. Bring to boil. Reduce heat; simmer uncovered 30 minutes, stirring occasionally.
Yield: 6 servings

🍎🍎🍎🍎🍎

Per serving: 298 Calories; 1g Fat (satfat 0.2g); 19g Protein; 55g Carbohydrate; 0mg Cholesterol; 1028mg Sodium

Refried Beans

1	pound dried pinto beans or black beans
5	cups water
3/4	cup chopped onion
2	cloves garlic, chopped
1	tablespoon chili powder
1	tablespoon ground cumin
1/2	teaspoon pepper
1/4	teaspoon salt

Sort and wash beans; place in a large Dutch oven. Cover with water to 2 inches above beans, and bring to a boil; cook 2 minutes. Remove from heat; cover and let stand 1 hour.

Drain beans, and return to pan. Add 5 cups water, onion, and garlic; bring to a boil. Cover, reduce heat, and simmer 2 hours or until tender.

Drain beans in a colander over a bowl, reserving 1-1/2 cups cooking liquid. Combine reserved cooking liquid, chili powder, cumin, pepper, and salt in pan. Add half of beans, and mash. Stir in remaining beans; cook over medium-low heat 5 minutes or until thickened, stirring occasionally.
Yield: 5 cups or 10 1/2-cup servings

Per serving: 165 Calories; 1g Fat (satfat 0.1g); 10g Protein; 31g Carbohydrate; 0mg Cholesterol; 70mg Sodium

South Seas Corn

3	cups frozen corn
1	clove garlic, minced
3	tablespoons unsweetened pineapple juice
3	tablespoons skim milk or soy milk
1 1/2	teaspoons soy sauce, low sodium
1/2	teaspoon honey
1/2	teaspoon cumin powder
1/4	teaspoon ginger
1/4	cup green onions, sliced

Coat a large skillet with cooking spray; place over medium heat until hot. Add corn and garlic; sauté 5 minutes. Combine pineapple juice, milk, soy sauce, honey, cumin, and ginger; add to corn. Cover, reduce heat, and simmer 5 minutes, stirring occasionally. Add green onions; cover and cook an additional 5 minutes.
Yield: 5 servings

Per serving: 101 Calories; 1g Fat (satfat 0.1g); 4g Protein; 24g Carbohydrate; 0mg Cholesterol; 57mg Sodium

Main Dishes

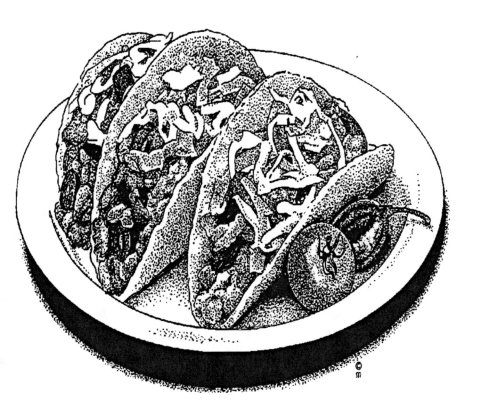

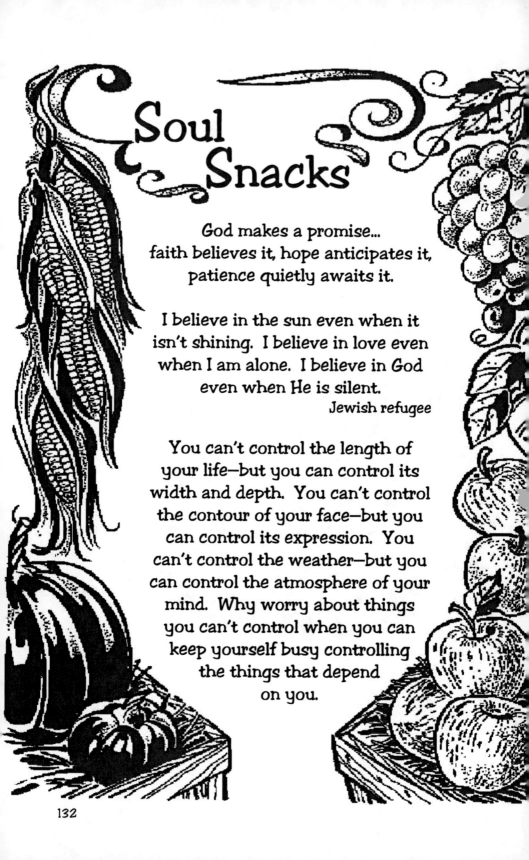

Soul Snacks

God makes a promise...
faith believes it, hope anticipates it,
patience quietly awaits it.

I believe in the sun even when it
isn't shining. I believe in love even
when I am alone. I believe in God
even when He is silent.

Jewish refugee

You can't control the length of
your life—but you can control its
width and depth. You can't control
the contour of your face—but you
can control its expression. You
can't control the weather—but you
can control the atmosphere of your
mind. Why worry about things
you can't control when you can
keep yourself busy controlling
the things that depend
on you.

Chicken Noodle Casserole

8	ounces wide noodles
1	each green pepper, seeded and diced
2	bunches green onions, chopped
1	tablespoon olive oil
2	cloves garlic, crushed
8	ounces sliced mushrooms
1	16-oz can tomato sauce
1	tablespoon chili powder
3	tablespoons dark brown sugar
4	ounces fat-free cream cheese *or* tofu
3	tablespoons Worcestershire sauce
1	teaspoon dry mustard
1 1/2	pounds chicken. skinned and boned
1	cup shredded lowfat Colby cheese *or* soy cheese
	salt and pepper to taste
3/4	cup Kraft Free® nonfat grated topping *or* soy Parmesan cheese

Cook the noodles according to package directions. Meanwhile, sauté the green pepper and green onions in the oil until softened. Add the garlic and mushrooms and continue cooking until limp. Add the tomato sauce, chili powder, sugar, cream cheese, Worcestershire sauce, mustard and sherry; simmer gently for 5 minutes.

Meanwhile, remove and discard skin from chicken; cut the meat into small pieces. Add to the sauce together with the grated cheese. Stir sauce into cooked noodles. Season to taste with salt and pepper. Pile mixture into a 9 by 13-inch pan and sprinkle with Parmesan cheese or grated topping. Bake at 350°F for 30 to 40 minutes or until bubbling.
Yield: 10 servings

Per serving: 273 Calories; 4g Fat (satfat 1.1g); 23g Protein; 31g Carbohydrate; 58mg Cholesterol; 512mg Sodium

Chuckwagon Beef and Pasta Skillet

2	cups Morningstar Farms®Harvest Burgers Recipe Crumbles *or* 1 pound lean ground beef
1	green bell pepper, chopped
1/2	cup onion, chopped
14	ounces fat-free beef broth
1	cup barbecue sauce
1/4	cup water
1/2	cup shredded lowfat Colby cheese *or* soy cheddar cheese
1 1/2	cups wagon wheel or rotini pasta, uncooked

In large nonstick skillet, put Crumbles or brown ground beef, bell pepper and onion over medium heat 6 minutes or until outside surface of beef is no longer pink, breaking beef up into 1/4 inch crumbles. Pour off drippings.

Stir in broth, pasta, barbecue sauce and water; bring to boil. Reduce heat to medium-low; cover and simmer 10-15 minutes or until pasta is almost tender. Uncover skillet; continue cooking 5-7 minutes or until pasta is tender and sauce is thickened, stirring occasionally. Sprinkle with cheese before serving.
Yield: 4-6 servings

🍎🍎🍎🍎🍎

Per serving: 252 Calories; 3g Fat (satfat 0.9g); 19g Protein; 37g Carbohydrate; 3mg Cholesterol; 879mg Sodium

Hoopla Chicken Lasagna

1	pound lasagna noodles, cooked & drained
1	cup onions, chopped
2	cloves garlic chopped
2	tablespoons margarine
1	recipe Mike's Spaghetti Sauce (p. 146) or 1 jar of spagetti sauce
1/2	cup water
4	ounces chopped green chilies, drained
1	teaspoon ground cumin
8	ounces fat-free cream cheese or tofu, silken
2	teaspoons chicken bouillon
3	cups chicken, chopped & cooked
4	cups shredded nonfat mozzarella cheese
3/4	cup celery, chopped

Preheat oven to 375° F. In Dutch oven, over medium heat, cook onion and garlic in margarine until tender. Stir in pasta sauce, water, chilies and cumin. Bring to a boil; reduce heat and simmer 10 minutes. In bowl, beat cream cheese with boullion until fluffy. Stir in chicken, 1-cup mozzarella and celery. On bottom of greased 15x9-inch baking dish, spread 3/4-cup sauce. Top with half each of the lasagna, chicken mixture, sauce and 1 1/2 cups mozzarella. Repeat layering, ending with sauce. Cover; bake 45 minutes, or until hot and bubbly. Uncover. Top with remaining 1 1/2-cups mozzarella. Bake 5 minutes longer. Refrigerate leftovers.
Yield: 12 -16 servings

Per serving: 313 Calories; 5g Fat (satfat 1.2); 29g Protein; 34g Carbohydrate; 42mg Cholesterol; 619mg Sodium

Main Dishes

Macaroni and Cheese with a Twist

1	pound vegetable twists, shells, rotini or elbow macaroni
2	tablespoons margarine *or* soy margarine
6	tablespoons unbleached flour
2	cups milk, skim
1	cup shredded lowfat cheddar cheese *or* soy cheddar cheese
1/2	cup lowfat cottage cheese
1/4	teaspoon cayenne pepper
1	teaspoon salt
1/2	cup Kraft Free® nonfat grated topping *or* soy Parmesan cheese

Prepare pasta according to package directions; drain and rinse under cold water. Set pasta aside. Heat oven to 375° F.

In medium saucepan, melt margarine over low heat. Stir in flour with a whisk and cook, stirring for 1 minute. Gradually whisk in the milk; bring the sauce to a boil, stirring constantly. Remove from heat and add Cheddar cheese, cayenne pepper and salt. Stir until cheese has melted.

In a large mixing bowl, stir the cheese sauce and pasta together. Spoon into a 1 1/2-quart ovenproof casserole dish. Sprinkle the Parmesan cheese over the top. Bake in a 375° F oven until browned on top and hot all the way through, about 30 to 35 minutes.

Yield: 6-8 servings

Variations on a Theme

VARIATION 1: Melt 2 tablespoons margarine in a large skillet. Add 1-cup dry bread crumbs; sauté until lightly toasted. Sprinkle breadcrumbs over casserole before baking.

VARIATION 2: Stir 1 cup frozen vegetables, such as peas, corn, lima beans or succotash, into the cheese sauce.

VARIATION 3: Stir two diced tomatoes and 2 tablespoons canned, chopped jalapenos into the cheese sauce.

VARIATION 4: Add 1 cup cottage cheese, 1/2 cup low-fat sour cream or 1/2 cup yogurt to the cheese sauce.

VARIATION 5: Add 1 tablespoon chopped fresh herbs, or 1/2 teaspoon dried, such as thyme, oregano, savory or basil, and 2 tablespoons chopped fresh parsley to the cheese sauce.

🍎🍎🍎🍎🍎

Per serving: 463 Calories; 5g Fat (satfat 1.7g); 22g Protein; 73g Carbohydrate; 6mg Cholesterol; 805mg Sodium

Mushrooms and Chicken Alfredo

8   ounces pasta fettuccini
2   tablespoons olive oil, divided
1   pound chicken, skinned, boned and cubed
12   ounces sliced mushrooms
1   recipe Alfredo sauce (p. 157)
1   cup peas optional
        chopped parsley for garnish, optional

Cook fettuccine according to package directions; drain. In a large nonstick skillet heat 1 tablespoon of the oil over high heat. Add chicken; cook and stir until golden on all sides, about 5 minutes; remove to a plate.

Heat remaining 1-tablespoon oil in the skillet. Add mushrooms; sauté until lightly browned, and liquid has evaporated, about 5 minutes. Reduce heat to medium-low; return chicken to skillet; stir in Alfredo sauce and 1 cup peas. If desired; cover and simmer until sauce is hot, about 3 minutes; stirring occasion-ally. Serve over fettuccine, sprinkled with parsley, if desired.
Yield 6 servings

🍎🍎🍎🍎🍎

Per serving: 290 Calories; 7g Fat (satfat 1.1g); 22g Protein; 35g Carbohydrate; 36mg Cholesterol; 85mg Sodium

Chicken Broccoli Casserole

4   chicken breasts without skin, cubed
3   cups instant rice
4   cups water, very hot
10   ounces chopped broccoli, frozen
1/2   cup shredded sharp cheddar cheese *or* soy cheddar cheese
2   cans 98% fat-free cream of chicken soup
3/4   cup plain nonfat yogurt *or* light sour cream
2   tablespoons lemon juice
2   teaspoons curry powder

Cook chicken until tender, about 1 hour. Cut into pieces. Place uncooked rice in 9x13 cake pan, add water and stir. Let sit while preparing sauce. Cook and drain broccoli. Layer rice, then chicken, then broccoli. Put grated cheese on broccoli.

SAUCE: Mix together soup, mayonnaise, lemon juice and curry powder, spread on top. Bake in 350° oven for 1 hour.
Yield: 12 servings

🍎🍎🍎🍎🍎

Per serving: 220 Calories; 3g Fat (satfat 1.5g); 22g Protein; 24g Carbohydrate; 50mg Cholesterol; 237mg Sodium

Tuna Pasta Salad
"Are you sure this is lowfat?
I could eat the whole thing myself IT IS SO GOOD!"
Bruce, kitchen tester

1	7 ounce package pasta shells, cooked & drained
6	ounces tuna in water, drained & flaked
1	large carrot, shredded
1	medium tomato, diced
1	stalk celery, diced
1/4	cup onion, chopped
3/4	cup plain lowfat yogurt or tofu
1	tablespoon lemon juice
2	teaspoons prepared mustard
1	teaspoon fresh dill weed, snipped
1/2	teaspoon salt
1/8	teaspoon pepper

In a large salad bowl, combine pasta, tuna, carrot and onion. Combine yogurt, lemon juice, mustard, dill weed, salt and pepper; whisk until smooth. Pour over pasta mixture; toss to coat. Cover and refrigerate for 1-2 hours.
Yield: 6 -8 servings.

🍎🍎🍎🍎🍎

Per serving: 129 Calories; 1g Fat (satfat 0.6g); 11g Protein; 18g Carbohydrate; 10mg Cholesterol; 351mg Sodium

Amazing Crustless Quiche

2 1/4	cups evaporated skim milk
3	eggs or 1/4 cup tofu
4	egg whites
1/2	cup unbleached flour
2	teaspoons onion flakes
1/4	teaspoon marjoram, dried and crushed
3/4	cup shredded Monterey jack cheese
1/3	cup Parmesan cheese or soy parmesan cheese
4	slices Canadian bacon, diced

Spray a 10-inch pie plate or quiche pan with vegetable spray. In blender combine milk, eggs, flour onion, marjoram, and a dash of salt. Cover; blend 15 seconds. Pour into pie plate. Dice up 4 slices of Canadian bacon and sprinkle over egg mix. Top with cheeses. Bake in a 400° F oven for 20 to 25 minutes or till a knife inserted near-center comes out clean. Let stand 5 minutes.
Yield: 8 -10 slices

🍎🍎🍎🍎🍎

Per serving: 194 Calories; 7g Fat (satfat 3.5); 17g Protein; 15g Carbohydrate; 89mg Cholesterol; 448mg Sodium

Baked Lentils

2	cups dried lentils
1/2	cup onions, diced
1/2	cup celery, diced
1/2	cup carrots, chopped
1/2	cup mushrooms, chopped
1	tablespoon olive oil
3	tablespoons flour
2	cups fat-free chicken broth or vegetarian broth
1/4	teaspoon basil
1/4	teaspoon ground thyme
1	tablespoon fresh parsley, chopped
	salt and pepper to taste
1/4	cup bread crumbs

Cook lentils in a quart of boiling water until barely tender, about 30 minutes. Drain.

While lentils are cooking, sauté vegetables in margarine over low heat until tender. Stir in flour and cook one minute, stirring constantly. Whisk in beef stock and bring sauce to a boil. Remove from heat and season to taste with salt, pepper, and herbs.

When lentils are cooked, drain and stir into sauce. Spread in a shallow, buttered pan. Sprinkle with breadcrumbs. Cut bacon slices into quarters and place on top of lentils.

Bake at 375°F for 40 minutes, until bacon browns.

Yields: 6 servings

🍎🍎🍎🍎🍎🍎

Per serving: 284 Calories; 3g Fat (satfat 0.5g); 23g Protein; 46g Carbohydrate; 0mg Cholesterol; 271mg Sodium

Main Dishes

Brown Rice Taco Stack Up

2 1/2	cups cooked brown rice
1/2	pound extra lean ground beef *or* veggie burger
1	teaspoon chili powder
3	cups Spanish tomato sauce
2	cups baked tortilla chips broken
1/2	cup green onion chopped
2	cups shredded lettuce
1	large tomatoes diced
1	cup shredded lowfat cheddar cheese, optional
	light sour cream, optional
	salsa, optional
	olives,optional

Brown meat with onion. Drain and rinse meat. Add oregano, and chili powder.
Mix well. Add tomato sauce, brown rice and water. Simmer until thickened. To
create a taco stack up break up a few tortilla chips on your plate. Then layer
rice mix, lettuce, tomato, olives, sour cream, salsa and cheese.
Yield: 6 - 8 servings

🍎🍎🍎🍎🍎

Per serving: 590 Calories; 10g Fat (satfat 3.0g); 19g Protein; 100g Carbohydrate; 23mg Cholesterol; 884mg Sodium

Carrot-Rice Bake

4	cups water
1	tablespoon chicken bouillon or vegetarian bouillon
1/2	teaspoon salt
2	cups carrots, chopped
1 1/2	cups brown rice
2	tablespoons margarine
1/2	teaspoon thyme crushed
1/2	cup sharp cheddar cheese *or* soy cheddar cheese

In saucepan bring water, bouillon, and salt to boiling. Stir in carrots, rice, butter,
and thyme; return to boiling. Turn mixture into a two-quart casserole dish. Bake,
covered at 325° for 25 minutes; stir. Sprinkle with cheese. Bake, uncovered
about 5 minutes longer. Garnish with parsley, if desired.
Yield: 8 servings

🍎🍎🍎🍎🍎

Per serving: 186 Calories; 5g Fat (satfat 2.1g); 5g Protein; 30g Carbohydrate;
7mg Cholesterol; 228mg Sodium

Spanish Rice

2	cups cooked rice
1/2	pound extra lean ground beef *or* Morningstar Farms® Harvest Burger Recipe Crumbles
16	ounces tomato sauce
1/4	cup onion chopped
1/2	cup green pepper, diced
1/2	teaspoon salt
1	clove garlic, minced
1	teaspoon chili powder
1	teaspoon Italian Seasoning or Herbes de Provence
1	cup salsa

Brown meat with the onion, and green pepper. Add tomato sauce, salsa, salt, garlic, chili powder and Italian Seasoning, mix well. Let simmer for about 15 to 20 minutes. Pour sauce over rice and mix well.   *Yield: 8 servings*

🍎🍎🍎🍎🍎

Per serving: 257 Calories; 5g Fat (satfat 2.1g); 10g Protein; 42g Carbohydrate; 20mg Cholesterol; 521mg Sodium

Mexican Meatloaf

1	tablespoon flax seed eggs or 1 egg
1/2	cup taco sauce
2	cups Cheese & Garlic Croutons, crushed
4	green onions, sliced
3/4	pound ground turkey or extra lean ground beef
15	ounces chili beans in sauce, spicy
1/3	cup shredded lowfat cheddar cheese or soy cheddar cheese
1	cup shredded lettuce
1	large tomato, diced
	light sour cream or soy yogurt
	salsa
	sliced olives, optional

In a bowl combine egg and taco sauce. Stir in crushed croutons and mix well. Add the ground beef mix well. Press into bottom of a 10x6x2-inch baking dish. Bake in a 350° F oven for 20 minutes. Drain off the fat. While the crust is cooking combine undrained chili beans, 1/2 cup shredded cheddar cheese, and green onions. Pour over meat mixture. Bake an additional 20 minutes or until meat is done and bean mixture is heated through. Cut into 6 servings. Place serving of meat on a bed of lettuce and tomatoes. Add a dollop of sour cream and salsa. Sprinkle with cheese.   *Yield: 8 servings*

🍎🍎🍎🍎🍎

Per serving: 138 Calories; 5g Fat (satfat 1.3g); 11g Protein; 11g Carbohydrate; 35mg Cholesterol; 178mg Sodium

Main Dishes

Chili Tamale Pie

1 1/4	cups Masa Harina
2/3	cup water
2	tablespoons canola oil
3/4	teaspoon salt
1	can Chili with sauce
1	can corn, drained
1	can, 4 oz. green chilies, drained
2	teaspoons chili powder
1/3	cup Masa Harina
2/3	cup shredded lowfat cheddar cheese

For crust: combine 1 1/4 cups of Masa Harina, 2/3 cup water, 2 tablespoons of oil and 3/4 teaspoons of salt in a 9 inch pie plate; mix well. Press evenly onto bottom and sides of pie plate.

For filling: combine remaining ingredients except cheese; pour into crust. Bake 375° oven about 25 minutes. Sprinkle with cheese; continue baking about 5 minutes. Let stand about 5 minutes: cut into wedges to serve.
Yield: 8 servings

🍎🍎🍎🍎🍎

Per serving: 209 Calories; 8.1g Fat (satfat 2.1g); 7.9g Protein; 26.3g Carbo-hydrate; 11mg Cholesterol; 545mg Sodium

Zucchini and Pasta

1	medium onion, finely chopped
1	tablespoon canola oil
1	20-oz. can crushed tomatoes
1	tablespoon basil
1	medium zucchini
1/2	pound whole wheat pasta shells
	pepper to taste
1/4	cup Parmesan cheese *or* soy parmesan cheese
2	tablespoons parsley, chopped

Sauté onions in oil until tender. Add tomatoes and sweet basil and simmer for 15 minutes. Slice zucchini and cut into 1/2-inch slices. Add remaining ingredients and cook until zucchini and pasta are tender and sauce is slightly thickened. Remove from heat and sprinkle with cheese and parsley.
Yield: 4 servings

🍎🍎🍎🍎🍎

Per serving: 298 Calories; 9g Fat (satfat 1.2g); 10g Protein; 49g Car-bohydrate; 4mg Cholesterol; 244mg Sodium

Fettuccini and Spinach

1/2	pound flat whole wheat noodles
1	tablespoon vegetable oil
1	clove garlic,crushed
3	cups spinach leaves, coarsely chopped
1/2	cup fat-free chicken broth *or* vegetable broth
1/4	cup Parmesan cheese *or* soy parmesan chees
1	cup lowfat cottage cheese or silken tofu
	pepper, to taste
1/2	teaspoon basil, dried
4	tablespoons parsley

Cook noodles in boiling water until tender. Drain. Meanwhile, heat the oil in a large skillet. Sauté the garlic and spinach for 2-3 minutes, stirring constantly and being careful not to burn the garlic. Add the broth, grated cheese, cottage cheese, pepper, and herbs. Stir and cook over low heat until blended (about 2 minutes). Toss cheese-spinach mixture with noodles. Turn onto a heated serving dish.
Yield: 5-6 servings

🍎🍎🍎🍎🍎

Per serving: 268 Calories; 7g Fat (satfat 1.4g); 15g Protein; 39g Carbohydrate; 5mg Cholesterol; 343mg Sodium

Seven Layer Dinner

1	pound lean chicken meat, cubed or lean ground beef
2	tablespoons fat-free chicken broth or oil
1	cup frozen corn
1	cup peas
1	cup green beans
1	cup potatoes, sliced
1	small onion, chopped
1	can tomato sauce
1	cup water

Cut chicken into cubes. In a skillet place chicken (or beef), broth and onion together, cook until chicken is done. In casserole dish put a layer of carrots, peas, corn, beans, potatoes, and meat. Top with tomato sauce and one cup water. Cook at 350°F about 30 minutes or until done.
Yield: 8 servings

🍎🍎🍎🍎🍎

Per serving: 119 Calories; 1g Fat (satfat 0.3g); 16g Protein; 12g Carbohydrate; 33mg Cholesterol; 296mg Sodium

Hawaiian Chicken

1	cup onions, chopped
2	tablespoons olive oil
1/4	cup unbleached flour
1 2/3	cups catsup
2	cups pineapple juice
1/2	cup brown sugar
1 1/3	tablespoons Worcestershire sauce
1	teaspoon garlic salt
1	teaspoon salt
1/2	teaspoon pepper
1/2	teaspoon cloves
3	pounds chicken breast halves without skin, cut into pieces

Sauté onion in margarine; stir in flour. Add catsup, pineapple juice, sugar, Worcestershire sauce, garlic salt, salt, pepper, and cloves. Cook, stirring constantly, until thickened. Place chicken in two-3 quart casseroles; pour half of sauce into each casserole. Bake at 350° for 1-1 1/2 hours or till done.
Yield: 8 servings

🍎🍎🍎🍎🍎

Per serving: 321 Calories; 5g Fat (satfat 1.0g); 33g Protein; 35g Carbohydrate; 79mg Cholesterol; 1057mg Sodium

Pepper Steak

1	pound sirloin steak, trimmed and thinly sliced
1/2	cup soy sauce
1	stalk celery, diced
1	clove garlic, minced
2	green pepper, diced or slivered
1	medium onion, slivered
1	cup fat-free beef broth
8	ounces mushrooms, canned
1	tablespoon cornstarch or arrowroot
2	cups cooked brown rice

Cut steak into small cubes or strips and brown with soy sauce. Add celery, peppers, onions, mushrooms, beef broth, salt and pepper to taste and continue browning. Add cornstarch and mix until thickened. Serve hot over brown rice.
Yield: 8 servings

🍎🍎🍎🍎🍎

Per serving: 276 Calories; 3g Fat (satfat 1.1g); 19g Protein; 42g Carbohydrate; 35mg Cholesterol; 1103mg Sodium

Humble Pie

1	pound extra lean ground beef *or*
	Morningstar Farms® Harvest Burger Recipe Crumbles
1	each onion, diced
1	green pepper, diced
1	stalk celery, diced
1/2	teaspoon salt
	pepper
1	tablespoon Worcestershire sauce
1/2	teaspoon garlic powder
2	tablespoons unbleached flour
2	cups skim milk or soy milk
10	large potatoes, diced
2	tablespoons Molly McButter ®
1/2	cup shredded lowfat cheddar cheese

Fill a large pot with water and heat to boiling. Meanwhile scrub and dice(I leave the skins on unless they are tough) the potatoes. Drop into boiling water and cook about 10 minutes or until soft. Drain water from potatoes (save it for soup stock). Add 1-cup milk and Molly McButter to potatoes and whip until smooth. Season to taste and set aside. Should be thinner than normal mashed potatoes.

Brown ground beef with onion, green pepper, and celery. Crumble meat. After meat is browned move all the ingredients to one side, and add flour, salt, pepper, Worcestershire sauce, garlic powder and mix to a smooth paste using the drippings from the meat. Add 1-cup milk, and stir constantly, until you have nice gravy, then mix the meat mix into the gravy. Remove from the heat.

In a large baking bowl, spray cooking oil on the inside, then put a fairly thick layer of potatoes covering the inside of the bowl, then a layer of meat, then a layer of potatoes, ending with a layer of potatoes. Sprinkle cheese on top and bake in 350°F oven for about 20 minutes or until heated all the way through.
Yield: 12 servings

Per serving: 183 Calories; 7g Fat (satfat 2.9g); 11.4g Protein; 17.2g Carbohydrate; 28mg Cholesterol; 306mg Sodium

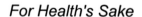

Main Dishes

Mike's Spaghetti Sauce

Serve over hot spaghetti, with a side order of French bread spread with Nicole's Favorite Herb and Garlic Cheese

1	medium onion, chopped
24	ounces tomato sauce
24	ounces water
2	tablespoons brown sugar
1	tablespoon chili powder
1	tablespoon salt
	dash pepper
	dash oregano
1	teaspoon Italian Seasoning or Herbes de Provence
1	green pepper, diced
1	4 oz can mushrooms
1	teaspoon garlic powder

Brown together meat and onion. Stir in the tomato sauce and water. Add the remaining ingredients and let simmer at least 2 hours to meld the seasonings. (You can add browned ground beef or Morningstar Farms® Harvest Burger Crumbles if you like meaty sauce)
Yield: 8 servings

Personal Note: I like to put it in my crock pot and simmer it all afternoon.

🍎🍎🍎🍎🍎

Per serving: 45 Calories; less than one gram Fat (satfat 0g); 2g Protein; 10g Carbohydrate; 0mg Cholesterol; 1396mg Sodium

Homestyle Macaroni and Cheese

1/4	pound whole wheat macaroni
2	cups shredded lowfat cheddar cheese
1 1/4	cups skim milk, hot
6	tablespoons bread crumbs *or* 3/4 cup fresh bread crumbs
1	medium onion, finely chopped
1	medium green pepper, chopped
1	teaspoon salt
2	teaspoons cornstarch *or* arrowroot
3	teaspoons water
	paprika
	parsley

Cook the macaroni in boiling salted water until it is tender but still firm. Drain it. Pour the hot milk over the breadcrumbs and cheese in a big bowl. Add the onion, lots of parsley, and the salt. Mix cornstarch with water till smooth, then mix in the macaroni. Put the mixture into a buttered casserole dish. Sprinkle it with paprika. Bake in a 350°F oven for about 30 minutes, or until the top of the macaroni and cheese is firm and golden brown.
Yield: 8 servings

Variation on a Theme
Just for fun replace the cheese with 1-cup mozzarella and 1 cup cheddar and a dash of cayenne pepper. What a stringy cheesy sensation this is.

🍎🍎🍎🍎🍎

Per serving: 168 Calories; 2.6g Fat (satfat 1.5g); 11g Protein; 19g Carbohydrate; 7mg Cholesterol; 565mg Sodium

Sweet And Sour Pork

*Leave out the meat and ladle this sassy dish into a
bowl of sweet and sour soup. Tasty!*

1 1/2	pounds pork sirloin, boneless, cubed
1	tablespoon canola oil
2	each peppers, sliced chunky
4	stalks celery, sliced
1	can pineapple chunks or tidbits
1	can mushrooms
1	20-oz. can stewed tomatoes
3	tablespoons cornstarch or arrowroot
1	teaspoon salt
1/2	teaspoon pepper
1/4	cup vinegar
1/2	cup lemon juice
2	tablespoons soy sauce
1 1/2	tablespoons cornstarch
1/2	cup honey
1	cup Pineapple juice
2	cups cooked rice

Place cornstarch, salt and pepper in plastic bag. Add cubed meat and shake
till meat is coated. Heat skillet or wok and add 1-tablespoon oil. When oil is
heated add meat. Cook quickly till crispy brown. Pour off any remaining oil.

To make sauce put vinegar, lemon juice, soy sauce, and honey in large
saucepan. Mix pineapple juice and cornstarch together into a smooth paste,
add to other ingredients and cook until you have a fairly thick sauce, stirring
constantly.

Add vegetables, pineapple, tomatoes, (squish tomatoes in your hand as you
add them), and meat. Simmer slightly. Vegetables should be fairly crisp. Add
meat. After sauce is thoroughly heated ladle over rice or Chinese noodles.
Side dishes could be broccoli with slivered almonds and raw cauliflower.

Yield 8 -10 servings

Variations on a Theme

Try this recipe with chicken or beef or better still meatless. To make sweet and
sour vegetables add 1 cup of snow peas, 1-cup broccoli flowerets and 1-cup
bean sprouts or any combination of your favorite vegetables

🍎🍎🍎🍎🍎

Per serving: 477 Calories; 8g Fat (satfat 2.2g); 23g Protein; 80g Carbohydrate;
54mg Cholesterol; 492mg Sodium

Pepperoni Potato Swirl

4	large potato
1/2	large onion, sliced
1	clove garlic
3	tablespoons Molly McButter® or 3 tablespoons margarine
3/4	cup skim milk, hot
1	egg or 1 flax seed egg
1/4	teaspoon black pepper
1/4	cup turkey pepperoni
1/2	cup shredded lowfat mozzarella cheese
1/3	cup green onions, chopped
1/4	cup Kraft Free® nonfat grated topping *or* soy parmesan cheese

Pare the potatoes. Cut into quarters. Cover with water. Add onion and garlic. Bring to a boil. Cover and simmer about 20 minutes or until just tender, not mushy. Drain. (Save potato water for soup). Mash potatoes. Add Molly McButter, milk, egg and black pepper. Whip until fluffy. Stir in pepperoni, cheese and green onions. Spoon into a greased ovenproof dish. Sprinkle with nonfat grated topping. Heat under a broiler until crusty or at 450°F for 5 minutes.

Yield: 4-6 servings

Variation on a Theme
Replace pepperoni with salami. If you're in a hurry try placing in microwave for 5 minutes on high.

🍎🍎🍎🍎🍎

Per serving: 194 Calories; 4g Fat (satfat 2.1g); 11g Protein; 26g Carbohydrate; 57mg Cholesterol; 752mg Sodium

Sassy Celery Casserole

4	cups celery thinly sliced
1/4	cup margarine
2	tablespoons unbleached flour
1/4	teaspoon salt
1	cup skim milk
3/4	cup shredded lowfat cheddar cheese or soy cheese
4	ounces canned mushrooms, drained
1/4	cup green pepper, chopped
1	teaspoon Italian seasoning or Herbes de Provence
1/4	teaspoon pepper
	dash garlic powder
1/4	cup onions, chopped
2	cups cooked rice

Cook celery, and onion, covered in butter till crisp-tender, about 15 minutes; stir in flour, salt, pepper, Italian seasoning, and garlic powder. Add milk; cook and stir till thickened and bubbly. Add 3/4 cup of cheese; stir until melted. Stir in mushrooms, and peppers. Turn into a 1-quart casserole. Bake uncovered at 350 for 20 minutes. Sprinkle with remaining 1/4-cup cheese. Serve over rice.

Yield: 6 servings

Per serving: 352 Calories; 6g Fat (satfat 1.9g); 10g Protein; 58g Carbohydrate; 4mg Cholesterol; 434mg Sodium

Tuna and Rice

2	cups cooked brown rice
1	large green pepper, chopped
2	stalks celery, chopped
1	small onion, diced
1/2	teaspoon Herbes de Provence or Italian Seasoning
1	clove garlic, minced
1	teaspoon dill weed
	dash cayenne pepper
	black pepper to taste
1	teaspoon lemon juice
1	can tuna in water
1	can 98% Fat Free Cream of Mushroom Soup

In a medium saucepan sauté onion, garlic, green pepper and celery in tuna water. Add tuna, soup, Herbes de Provence, cayenne pepper, pepper and lemon juice. Mix well and simmer till heated through. Pour sauce over rice and mix well. Serve with minted peas and fruit.
Yield 8 servings

🍎🍎🍎🍎🍎

Per serving: 213 Calories; 2g Fat (satfat 0.4g); 9g Protein; 39g Carbohydrate; 7mg Cholesterol; 251mg Sodium

Tuna Dressing

1	loaf bread, broken
2	cans tuna in water drained
2	each onions, diced
1	stalk celery, diced
2	tablespoons flax seed eggs or 2 eggs
1	teaspoon poultry seasoning
	salt and pepper to taste
2	cans 98% Fat Free Cream of Mushroom Soup
	hot water

Mix bread, tuna fish, onions, celery, 1 can of cream of mushroom soup and seasonings together. Add eggs and hot water until mixture is just moist. Put into a 9 x13-inch pan. Pour cream of mushroom soup over the top, Bake at 350 for 30-40 minutes.
Yield: 12 servings

🍎🍎🍎🍎🍎

Per serving: 171 Calories; 2.4g Fat (satfat 0.6g); 11.1g Protein; 25.4g Carbohydrate; 9mg Cholesterol; 571mg Sodium

Wheat Chili

2	cups wheat kernels
1	large onion
1	tablespoon chili powder
1	teaspoon oregano
20	oz. can crushed tomatoes
1	can black olives, chopped
1	pound Morningstar Farms® Harvest Burger Recipe Crumbles or extra lean ground beef
1/2	large green pepper
1	teaspoon garlic powder
1/2	teaspoon cayenne
2	cups tomato sauce

Soak wheat overnight in cold water. Simmer for an hour or so, drain off all but 1/2-cup water, brown ground beef, onion, and green pepper, add to wheat. Add remaining ingredients and stir well. Simmer 30 to 45 minutes. If desired, pour into a casserole dish, top with cheese, pop into oven till bubbly.
Yield: 8 servings

🍎🍎🍎🍎🍎

Per serving: 218 Calories; 1.6g Fat (satfat 0.3); 10.3g Protein; 45g Carbohydrate; 0mg Cholesterol; 599mg Sodium

Sauces and Dressings

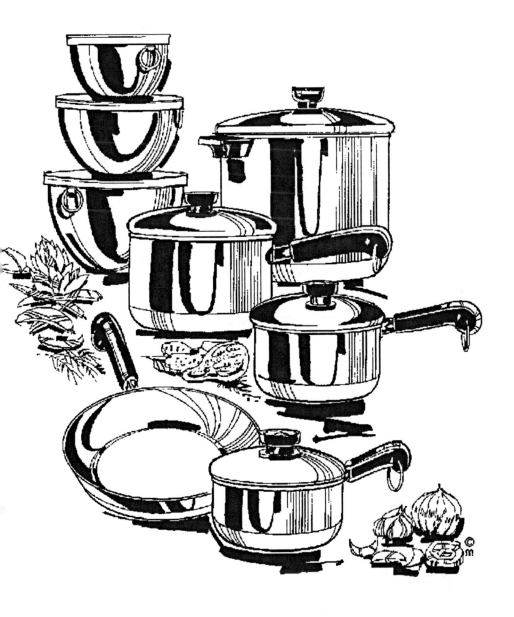

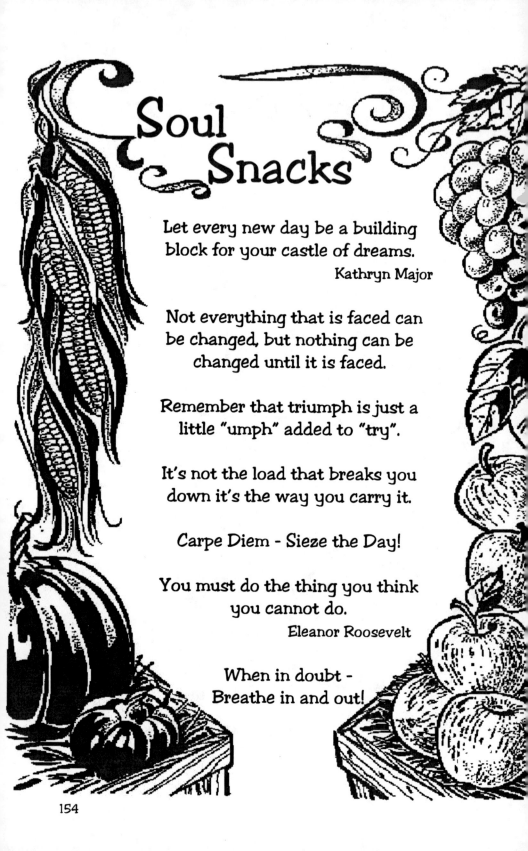

Soul Snacks

Let every new day be a building block for your castle of dreams.

Kathryn Major

Not everything that is faced can be changed, but nothing can be changed until it is faced.

Remember that triumph is just a little "umph" added to "try".

It's not the load that breaks you down it's the way you carry it.

Carpe Diem - Sieze the Day!

You must do the thing you think you cannot do.

Eleanor Roosevelt

When in doubt - Breathe in and out!

Alfredo Sauce

2	cloves garlic, minced
2	tablespoons Molly McButter®
1	cup silken tofu, soft
2	cups evaporated skim milk or soy milk
1	cup Parmesan cheese or soy Parmesan cheese
1/4	cup parsley, chopped
1/4	teaspoon salt
	pepper to taste

With a wire whisk mix together tofu, milk, Molly McButter® and garlic until smooth. Heat 1 minute over medium heat (do not boil). Blend in Parmesan cheese, parsley, salt and pepper. Cook until desired thickness is accomplished.
Yield: 4 cups

🍎🍎🍎🍎🍎

Per serving: 60 Calories; 2g Fat (satfat 1.0g); 5g Protein; 5g Carbohydrate; 5mg Cholesterol; 235mg Sodium

Basic White Sauce

2	tablespoons corn oil
2	tablespoons flour, unbleached
1	cup skim milk or soy milk
	salt and pepper, to taste

Pour oil into a saucepan over low heat. Blend in flour. Cook over low heat, stirring until mixture is smooth and bubbly. Remove from heat. Stir in milk. Heat to boiling, stirring constantly. Cook until desired thickness is achieved.
Yields: 1 cup (one serving is 2 tablespoons).

Variations on a Theme
Cheese Sauce (for vegetables, rice or macaroni) Prepare white sauce as directed. Stir in 1/4 teaspoon dry mustard and 1/2 cup shredded Cheddar cheese or cheddar soy cheese. Heat over low heat, stirring constantly, until cheese is melted and sauce is smooth.
Cucumber Sauce (for salmon and other fish) Stir in 1/2 cup shredded or thinly sliced cucumber and a of dash cayenne red pepper; simmer 5 minutes, stirring occasionally.
Curry Sauce (for chicken, shrimp and rice) Add 1/2-teaspoon curry powder with the flour.
Dill Sauce (for bland meat or fish). Add 1-teaspoon fresh or 1/2 teaspoon dried dill weed and dash nutmeg with flour.

🍎🍎🍎🍎🍎

Per serving: 48 Calories; 3g Fat (satfat 0.5g); 1g Protein; 3g Carbohydrate; 1mg Cholesterol; 16mg Sodium

Barbecue Sauce
This is a good basic recipe for chicken.

1	cup onion, finely chopped
1	cup ketchup, low sodium
1/4	cup brown sugar
1/4	cup apple cider vinegar
1/4	cup Worcestershire sauce
1	teaspoon dry mustard
1/4	teaspoon hot sauce
2	teaspoons salt
1	teaspoon lemon juice
	Pepper to taste

Mix all ingredients together. Keeps for one month in the refrigerator.
Yields 2 cups.

Variations on a Theme
for Pork, substitute 1 cup peach preserves for ketchup.

🍎🍎🍎🍎🍎

Per serving: 30 Calories; less than one gram of Fat (satfat 0g); 0.3g Protein;
8g Carbohydrate; 0mg Cholesterol; 349mg Sodium

Pizza Sauce

8	ounces tomato sauce
6	ounces tomato paste
2	teaspoons onion, minced
1/2	teaspoon dried basil
1/2	teaspoon dried oregano
1/2	teaspoon parsley, freeze-dried
1/4	teaspoon fennel seeds
1/4	teaspoon garlic powder

Mix ingredients in saucepan. Bring to boil. Cook over low heat about 10
minutes. Use approximately 3/4-cup sauce for each pizza. Store remainder
in refrigerator or freeze for future use.
Yields 1 3/4 cups.

🍎🍎🍎🍎🍎

Per serving: 28 Calories; less than one gram of Fat (satfat 0g); 1g Protein; 6g
Carbohydrate; 0mg Cholesterol; 189mg Sodium

Quickie Salsa

3	medium tomatoes, finely chopped
3	medium tomatillos, finely chopped
1	tablespoon onion minced
2	tablespoons cilantro, chopped
1	jalapeno pepper, seeded and minced
1/4	teaspoon cumin powder
1/4	teaspoon salt

In a medium bowl, mix together all ingredients. Serve right away with crisp chips for dipping or as a sauce over enchiladas, or cover and refrigerate up to 8 hours for best flavor and texture.
Yield: 8 servings

🍎🍎🍎🍎🍎

Per serving: 16 Calories; less than one gram Fat (satfat 0g); 1g Protein; 3g Carbohydrate; 0mg Cholesterol; 76mg Sodium

Shanni's Hot Fudge Sauce

1/2	cup margarine
2	cups fructose or natural sugar
1/2	teaspoon salt
1/2	cup cocoa powder
1	can evaporated skim milk
1	teaspoon vanilla

Place the cocoa powder, sugar, and salt in a medium mixing bowl. Slowly whisk in half of the milk until the mixture forms a thick paste. Whisk in the remaining half of the milk, and transfer the mixture to a small high-sided saucepan. Add the corn syrup, and stir to thoroughly combine.

Place the saucepan over medium-high heat. Cook the sauce, stirring occasionally with a wooden spoon, until the temperature registers 200° on a candy thermometer, 4 to 5 minutes. Remove the saucepan from the heat, and transfer the sauce to a small bowl to cool until lukewarm. Serve immediately by spooning the sauce over ice cream, etc.

Cooking the sauce to 200° gives it the consistency of a rich and thick hot-fudge topping. This sauce can also be served over nonfat frozen yogurt or used as syrup in skim milk mixed with club soda for a nonfat chocolate egg cream.
Yield: 3 cups (serving size 2 tablespoons)

🍎🍎🍎🍎🍎

Per serving: 60 Calories; 2g Fat (satfat 0.9g); 1g Protein; 11g Carbohydrate; 0mg Cholesterol; 65mg Sodium

Creamy Garlic Dressing

1	cup plain lowfat yogurt or silken tofu
3	tablespoons water
2	tablespoons cider vinegar
1	clove garlic, finely chopped
1/2	teaspoon honey
1/4	teaspoon salt
1/8	teaspoon pepper

In small bowl, stir together all ingredients until well blended. Cover and refrigerate for several hours.
Yield: 1 cup (one serving equals 2 tablespoons)

🍎🍎🍎🍎🍎

Per serving: 16 Calories; less than one gram Fat (satfat 0.2); 1g Protein; 2g Carbohydrate; 1mg Cholesterol; 69mg Sodium

Creamy Italian Dressing

1 1/4	teaspoons thyme
1/4	teaspoon basil
1/4	teaspoon oregano
5	ounces silken tofu, soft
1	clove garlic, minced
1	tablespoon olive oil
2	teaspoons red wine vinegar or apple cider vinegar
1	teaspoon onion, minced
	salt and freshly ground pepper

Combine herbs in mortar and pestle and crush until well blended. If you don't have a mortar and pestle, press between your fingers to release flavors. In a blender, combine herbs with remaining ingredients and mix until smooth, stopping to scrape down sides as necessary.
Yield: about 2/3 cup (serving size equals 2 tablespoons)

🍎🍎🍎🍎🍎

Per serving: 25 Calories; 2.5g Fat (satfat 0.3g); 0.4g Protein; 0.7g Carbohydrate; 0mg Cholesterol; 2mg Sodium

French-Honey Dressing

1	can tomato soup
1/4	cup vinegar
1/3	cup canola oil
1/3	cup water
1	tablespoon onion powder
3/4	teaspoon salt
1/2	teaspoon dry mustard
1	tablespoon Worcestershire sauce
1/2	teaspoon Herbes de Provence
1/4	cup honey

Put tomato soup, vinegar, oil and water in blender and mix well. Then add onion powder, salt, mustard, Worcestershire sauce, honey, and Herbes de Provence. Mix well. Store in jar with a tight lid in the refrigerator.
Yield: 2 cups (serving size is 2 tablespoons)

🍎🍎🍎🍎🍎

Per serving: 65 Calories; 5g Fat (satfat 0.3); 0g Protein; 6g Carbohydrate; 0mg Cholesterol; 165mg Sodium

Green Goddess Dressing

1	tablespoon apple cider vinegar
1/2	cup plain lowfat yogurt
1/2	cup light sour cream
3/4	cup buttermilk or soymilk + lemon juice
2	cloves garlic, minced
1/2	cup fresh chives, chopped
1/4	cup fresh parsley, chopped
1	tablespoon fresh tarragon, chopped
1	tablespoon fresh basil, chopped
2	tablespoons capers
	salt and pepper

In blender: begin by chopping herbs, capers, adding vinegar as herbs are chopped. Blend in yogurt and sour cream. Slowly add buttermilk while blending, until desired consistency is reached.
Yield 2 cups (serving size is 2 tablespoons).

🍎🍎🍎🍎🍎

Per serving: 13 Calories; less than one gram Fat (satfat 0.1); 1g Protein; 1g Carbohydrate; 1mg Cholesterol; 29mg Sodium

Honey Mustard Dressing

1/2   **cup plain nonfat yogurt or soy yogurt**
1   **tablespoon cider vinegar**
2   **teaspoons Dijon mustard**
2   **teaspoons honey**
      salt and freshly ground pepper to taste

In a small bowl, whisk yogurt, vinegar, mustard, honey and salt until blended. Add a generous grinding of pepper and whisk again. (Alternatively, combine all ingredients in a small jar, secure the lid and shake until blended.)
Yield 2/3 cup (serving size 2 tablespoons)

🍎🍎🍎🍎🍎

Per serving: 19 Calories; less than one gram Fat (satfat 0g); 1g Protein; 4g Carbohydrate; 0mg Cholesterol; 35mg Sodium

Italian Dressing

2/3   **cup canola oil *or* olive oil**
1/4   **cup white vinegar**
1   **teaspoon minced garlic**
1/8   **cup Parmesan cheese or soy Parmesan cheese**
1/8   **teaspoon paprika**
1/2   **teaspoon fructose or natural sugar**
1/2   **teaspoon salt**
1/4   **teaspoon pepper**
1/2   **teaspoon celery leaves**
1   **teaspoon parsley**
1/4   **teaspoon dry mustard**

Place all ingredients in a small jar. Place lid on jar and shake vigorously. Keep in refrigerator.
Yield: 1 cup (serving size 2 tablespoons).

🍎🍎🍎🍎🍎

Per serving: 169 Calories; 19g Fat (satfat 1.5g); 1g Protein; 1g Carbohydrate; 1mg Cholesterol; 157mg Sodium

For Health's Sake

Lemon Fruit Salad Dressing

Sauces and Dressings

2   teaspoons cornstarch or arrowroot
1/4   cup water
6   ounces lemonade, frozen concentrate
2   cups fat-free whipped topping

Mix cornstarch and water together in small saucepan till smooth, add lemonade. Mix well and cook over low heat until thickened. Cool. When cooled fold in whipped topping.
Yield: 2 1/2 cups (serving size 2 tablespoons)

Variation on a Theme
This recipe is so simple you could use any flavor of frozen juice concentrate, like strawberry banana orange, now doesn't that sound scrumptious?

🍎🍎🍎🍎🍎

Per serving: 28 Calories; less than one gram Fat (satfat 0g); 0g Protein; 7g Carbohydrate; 0mg Cholesterol; 8mg Sodium

Ranch-Style Buttermilk Salad Dressing

1   cup buttermilk
1/2   cup plain nonfat yogurt or soy yogurt
3   tablespoons parsley, minced
3   tablespoons chives, chopped
1   clove garlic, minced
1   tablespoon tarragon, chopped
1   tablespoon lemon juice
1/2   tablespoon Worcestershire sauce
       salt and pepper to taste

Mix all ingredients together. Cover and chill.
Yield: 1 1/2 cups (serving size is 2 tablespoons).

🍎🍎🍎🍎🍎

Per serving: 19 Calories; less than one gram Fat (satfat 0.1g); 2g Protein; 3g Carbohydrate; 1mg Cholesterol; 40mg Sodium

Sweet Treats

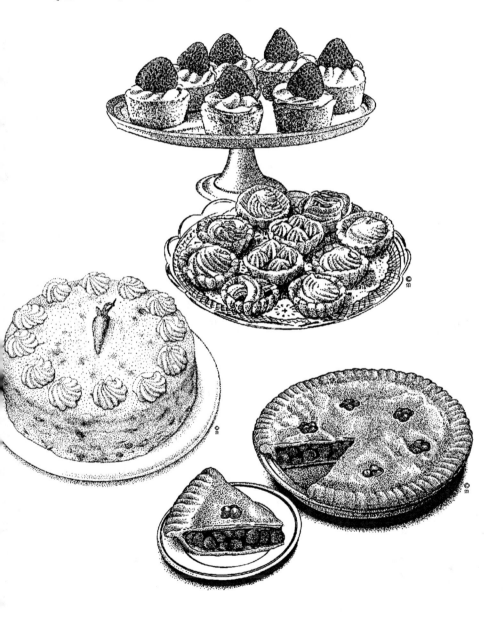

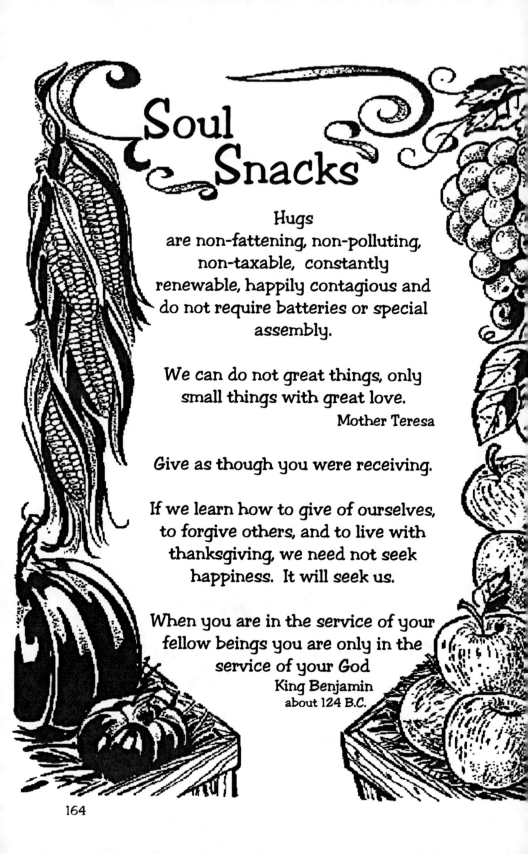

Soul
Snacks

Hugs
are non-fattening, non-polluting,
non-taxable, constantly
renewable, happily contagious and
do not require batteries or special
assembly.

We can do not great things, only
small things with great love.
Mother Teresa

Give as though you were receiving.

If we learn how to give of ourselves,
to forgive others, and to live with
thanksgiving, we need not seek
happiness. It will seek us.

When you are in the service of your
fellow beings you are only in the
service of your God
King Benjamin
about 124 B.C.

A.B.C.Brownies

1/2	cup applesauce, unsweetened
2	tablespoons margarine, softened
2/3	cup brown sugar, packed
1	egg, beaten or 1 flax seed egg
1	teaspoon vanilla
1 1/4	cups unbleached flour
1/3	cup wheat germ
1/4	cup almonds, toasted and chopped
1/4	cup chocolate chips

Mix applesauce, margarine, brown sugar, eggs and vanilla together till smooth. Set aside. In another bowl, combine flour, wheat germ and baking powder. Stir in sugar and egg mixture. Pour batter into a greased 8-inch square pan. Sprinkle with almonds and chocolate chips. Bake at 375°F for 20 minutes. Cut brownies when slightly cooled. *Yield: 16 2-inch squares (serving size 1 square)*

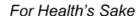

Per serving: 100 Calories; 3g Fat (satfat 0.8g); 2g Protein; 17g Carbohydrate; 11mg Cholesterol; 19mg Sodium

Applesauce-Spice Cookies

1/2	cup margarine
1/2	cup brown sugar or honey
1/3	cup fructose or natural sugar
1	flax seed eggs or 1 egg
2	cups unbleached flour
1/2	teaspoon cinnamon
1/4	teaspoon cloves
1/2	teaspoon salt
1/2	teaspoon baking soda
1	teaspoon baking powder
1	cup applesauce, thick unsweetened

Cream margarine and sugars together. Beat egg, add to creamed mixture and blend well. Sift all dry ingredients together and add alternately with the applesauce to the creamed mixture. Be sure to add flour first and last. Drop on well-greased cookie sheet. Bake 15 minutes at 375° F.

Yield: 2 1/2 dozen large cookies (serving size 1 cookie)
Variation on a Theme
Add 1 cup chopped nuts, dates or raisins to the batter. Before baking, top each cookie with a red or green cherry and brush tops with Cream Cheese Spread.

🍎🍎🍎🍎🍎

Per serving: 67 Calories; 2g Fat (satfat 0.4g); 1g Protein; 11g Carbohydrate; 0mg Cholesterol; 97mg Sodium

Basic Sugar Cookies

3	tablespoons margarine, softened
2/3	cup fructose
1	flax seed eggs or 1 egg
1	tablespoon lemon juice
1 1/2	cups all-purpose flour
1/2	teaspoon baking soda
1/4	teaspoon nutmeg
2	tablespoons fructose

Cream softened margarine; gradually add 2/3-cup fructose, beating at medium speed of an electric mixer until well blended. Add egg and lemon juice; beat well.

Combine flour, baking soda, and nutmeg; gradually add to creamed mixture, beating well.

Shape dough into 26 balls; roll in remaining 2 tablespoons sugar. Place 2 inches apart on ungreased cookie sheets, and pat each portion into a 2-inch circle. Bake at 375°F for 9 minutes. Cool on wire racks.
Yield: 26 cookies (serving size 1 cookie)

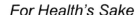

Per serving: 52 Calories; 1g Fat (satfat 0.2g); 1g Protein; 10g Carbohydrate; 0mg Cholesterol; 36mg Sodium

Caramel Sour Cream Cookies

1/2	cup applesauce, unsweetened
1/2	cup brown sugar
1	egg *or* 1 flax seed egg
1/2	cup sour cream, light *or* soy sour cream
2 1/4	cups unbleached flour
1/4	teaspoon salt
1 1/2	teaspoons baking powder
1/4	teaspoon baking soda
1/2	teaspoon nutmeg
	fructose or Natural sugar

Cream applesauce and sugar. Add beaten egg to sour cream. Sift flour, salt, baking powder, soda, and nutmeg together. Add alternately with egg mixture to the creamed oil and sugar. Chill thoroughly. Use a rolling pin stocking and pastry cloth and roll only a small portion at a time to 1/4-inch thickness. Sprinkle with fructose and bake on a greased cookie sheet 15 minutes at 350°F.
Yield: 4 dozen 2-inch cookies (serving size 1 cookie)

🍎🍎🍎🍎🍎

Per serving: 30 Calories; less than one gram Fat (satfat 0g); 1g Protein; 6g Carbohydrate; 4mg Cholesterol; 31mg Sodium

Chinese Chews

2	eggs *or* 2 flax seed eggs
2/3	cup brown sugar
3/4	cup unbleached flour
1	teaspoon baking powder
1/4	teaspoon salt
1	cup dates finely chopped
1/2	cup pecans, roasted and chopped

Beat eggs and add to sugar. Sift all dry ingredients together and mix in dates and nuts. Add flour mixture to sugar mixture. Beat well. Line a 6x11-inch pan with waxed paper and spread dough in it to depth of 1/2 inch. Bake 40 minutes at 350° F. *Yield: 22 1x3-inch bars*

🍎🍎🍎🍎🍎

Per serving: 66 Calories; 1g Fat (satfat 0.2g); 1g Protein; 13g Carbohydrate; 16mg Cholesterol; 48mg Sodium

Cookie Sheet Cake

1	cup water
1 1/2	cups raisins
1/4	cup margarine
1/4	cup plain lowfat yogurt
3/4	cup brown sugar
1	egg or 2 tablespoons tofu
1	tablespoon vanilla
2	cups unbleached flour
1	teaspoon cinnamon
1 1/2	teaspoon baking soda
1	teaspoon salt
1/2	cup walnuts, toasted and finely chopped

Boil the cup of water and the raisins for 10 minutes then save 3/4 of a cup of the raisin water. Cream the butter and the sugar. Then mix in the remaining ingredients. Make sure to add the raisins and the 3/4 of a cup of raisin water to the mix. Pour onto a greased cookie sheet. Bake at 350° for 25 minutes. When cool frost with white frosting and sprinkle with coconut, and or dust with coconut dust. You can make this by putting the coconut into a smaller grinder and grinding it until it becomes a fine powder.
Yield: 36 squares (serving size 1 bar)

Per serving: 68 Calories; 1g Fat (satfat 0.3g); 1g Protein; 13g Carbohydrate; 5mg Cholesterol; 110mg Sodium

Date Honeys

3	eggs *or* 3 flax seed eggs
1	cup honey, strained
1 1/2	cups unbleached flour
1	teaspoon salt
2	cups dates, ground
1	cup walnuts, chopped

Beat eggs until thick and combine with honey. Sift the flour, baking powder and salt together and add to eggs and honey. Add dates and nuts. Combine all ingredients and pour only to 1/4-inch depth, into two 7x11-inch pans which have been lined with waxed paper. Bake in a moderate oven (350°) 40 minutes. Remove from pan and cool. Cut into 22 bars 1 inch wide or wrap the whole cake in waxed paper and store until ready to cut. Honey cookies can be kept 2 or 3 weeks and the flavor will improve.
Yield: 22 bars (serving size 1 bar)

Per serving: 135 Calories; 1g Fat (satfat 0.2g); 2g Protein; 30g Carbohydrate; 25mg Cholesterol; 105mg Sodium

Honey Hermits

2 1/2	cups flour
1	teaspoon baking soda
1/4	teaspoon salt
1/2	teaspoon allspice
1/2	teaspoon cinnamon
1/2	cup margarine or soy margarine
1	cup honey
1/3	cup brown sugar
2	egg whites or 1 flax seed egg
3	tablespoons skim milk or soy milk
1	cup seedless raisins
1	cup dried currants
1	cup dates chopped
1/2	cup walnuts, toasted and chopped

Sift flour, soda, salt and spices together 3 times. Cream margarine with honey and sugar. Add eggs. Add milk, dry ingredients, fruit and nuts and mix thoroughly. Drop from teaspoon onto greased cookie sheet and bake at 400°F. 10 to 12 minutes.

Yield: 4 dozen cookies (serving size 1 cookie)

🍎🍎🍎🍎🍎

Per serving: 91 Calories; 1g Fat (satfat 0.3g); 1g Protein; 19g Carbohydrate; 0mg Cholesterol; 58mg Sodium

Luscious Apricot Squares

2/3	cup apricots, dried
1/2	cup plain lowfat yogurt or tofu
1 1/3	cups unbleached flour
1	teaspoon baking powder
1/4	cup fructose
1/4	teaspoon salt
1/2	cup brown sugar, packed
3	egg whites or 3 unflavored gelatin eggs
1/2	cup fructose
1/2	teaspoon vanilla
1/2	cup walnuts, toasted and chopped

Rinse apricots. Cover with water; boil 10 minutes. Drain; cool; chop finely.
Start heating oven to 350°. Grease 8-inch square pan. Mix yogurt, 1/4-cup
fructose and 1 cup sifted flour until crumbly. Pack this mixture into cake pan.
Bake about 25 minutes, or until lightly browned. Sift together 1/3-cup flour,
baking powder, and salt. With electric mixer at medium speed gradually beat
1/2 cup fructose into egg whites; then beat in flour mixture, vanilla, walnuts, and
apricots. Spread over baked layer, then bake 30 minutes or until done. Cool
in pan, on wire rack; then cut into squares, store tightly covered.
Yield: 16 squares (serving size 1 square)

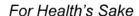

Per serving: 80 Calories; 1g Fat (satfat 0.1g); 2g Protein; 16g Carbohydrate;
0mg Cholesterol; 62mg Sodium

Sweet Treats

Easy Does It Cookie Bars

These familiar tasting cookie bars are similar to 7 Layer or Magic Cookie Bars but have half the fat and carbohydrates of our old favorites.

1/2	cup margarine or soy margarine
1 1/4	cups graham cracker crumbs
1	can fat free sweetened condensed milk
1	cup chocolate chips
1	cup butterscotch chips
1/2	cup walnuts, toasted and chopped
1 1/2	cups coconut

Preheat oven to 350. Spray 13x9-inch baking pan with cooking spray. In a bowl mix crumbs and margarine. When crumbs are thoroughly mixed pat into bottom of baking pan. Pour sweetened condensed milk evenly over crumbs. Top evenly with chocolate chips, butterscotch chips, coconut and nuts; press down gently. Bake 25 minutes or until lightly browned. Cool thoroughly before cutting. Loosely cover any leftovers. *Yield: 32 2 1/2-inch squares.(serving size 1 square)*

🍎🍎🍎🍎🍎🍎

Per serving: 124 Calories; 5g Fat (satfat 2g); 2g Protein; 19g Carbohydrate; 1mg Cholesterol; 61mg Sodium

Moist and Chewy Brownies

1/3	cup applesauce
2	tablespoons margarine or soy margarine
3/4	cup natural sugar or fructose
1	teaspoon vanilla
2	flax seed eggs *or* 2 egg whites + 1 egg
1/2	cup unbleached flour
1/3	cup cocoa powder
1/4	teaspoon salt
1/2	teaspoon baking powder
1/2	cup chopped walnuts (optional)
	Vegetable cooking spray

Blend applesauce, margarine, sugar and vanilla in a mixing bowl. Add eggs; beat well with spoon. Combine flour, cocoa, baking powder and salt; gradually add to egg mixture until well blended. Stir in nuts. Spread into a 9-inch square pan. Bake at 350° for 20 to 25 minutes or until brownie begins to pull away from edges of pan. Cool in pan. Frost if desired; cut into squares.
Yield: 16 brownies (serving size 1 brownie)

🍎🍎🍎🍎🍎🍎

Per serving: 73 Calories; 2g Fat (satfat 0.4g); 1g Protein; 15g Carbohydrate; 0mg Cholesterol; 58mg Sodium

Myndy's Chocolate Chip Cookies

1/2	cup applesauce
3/4	cup brown sugar
3	flax seed eggs *or* 2 egg hites + 1 egg
1	teaspoon vanilla
1	cup cooked whole wheat natural cereal or cooked oatmeal
1/2	cup plain nonfat yogurt
2 1/4	cups whole wheat flour
1	teaspoon baking soda
1/2	teaspoon salt
1 1/2	cups chocolate chips
3/4	cup walnuts, toasted and chopped
3/4	cup sunflower seeds, toasted

Cream the butter and the sugar or honey. Add the eggs and beat until fluffy. Add vanilla, cooked rolled wheat cereal and the yogurt and continue to mix. Then stir together the flour, soda, and the salt. This batter will seem more like a cake batter to you than cookie dough, but this is what makes the cookies moist and light. Do not add additional flour. Now add the chocolate or carob chips, one of the above mentioned nuts, and the sunflower seeds. Mix well. Drop by a teaspoon onto a cookie sheet. Bake for 10 minutes at 375. If you want a harder cookie increase the baking time by 2 to 5 minutes.

Note: If you use salted sunflower seeds you may wish to delete the 1/2-tea-spoon of salt that is called for in this recipe.

Yield: 5 dozen cookies (serving size 1 cookie)

🍎🍎🍎🍎🍎

Per serving: 58 Calories; 2g Fat (satfat 0.8g); 1g Protein; 10g Carbohydrate; 0mg Cholesterol; 42mg Sodium

Oatmeal Raisin Cookies

1/2	cup margarine
1/4	cup applesauce
2/3	cup brown sugar packed
2/3	cup Natural sugar or fructose
1	egg *or* 2 tablespoons tofu
1/4	cup water
1	teaspoon vanilla
1	cup unbleached flour
1/2	teaspoon salt
1	teaspoon cinnamon
1/2	teaspoon baking soda
1/2	teaspoon cloves
1	cup raisins
1/2	cup walnuts, toasted and chopped
3	cups quick-cooking oats

Heat oven to 350°F. Mix thoroughly margarine, applesauce, sugars, egg, water and vanilla. Stir in remaining ingredients.

Drop dough by rounded teaspoons 1 inch apart onto greased baking sheet. Bake 12 to 15 minutes or until almost no imprint remains when touched with finger. Immediately remove from baking sheet. Store in tightly covered container. Makes about 5 dozen cookies.
Yield: 5 dozen cookies (serving size 1 cookie)

Variation on a Theme
Banana Oatmeal Cookies: Omit water, increase soda to 1 teaspoon and stir in 1 cup mashed banana (2 to 3 medium) into margarine mixture.

🍎🍎🍎🍎🍎

Per serving: 54 Calories; 1g Fat (satfat 0.3g); 1g Protein; 9g Carbohydrate; 3mg Cholesterol; 44mg Sodium

Peanut Butter Crisscrosses

If you love peanut butter cookies you will find these fit the bill and with
reduce fat peanut butter you get more flavor and less fat.

1/2	cup margarine or soy margarine
1/2	cup plain nonfat yogurt or soy yogurt
1/2	cup brown sugar
1	teaspoon vanilla
3	cups unbleached flour
2	teaspoons baking soda
1/2	teaspoon salt
1/4	cup honey
2	egg whites or 2 flax seed eggs
3/4	cup peanut butter, reduced fat

Thoroughly cream shortening, sugars, eggs, and vanilla. Stir in peanut butter. Sift dry ingredients; stir into creamed mixture. Drop by rounded teaspoon or ungreased cookie sheet. Press with fork to make crisscross. Bake in moderate oven (350) about 10 minutes.

Yield: 5 dozen cookies (serving size 1 cookie)
*For richer cookies, use 2 cups flour.

Per serving: 61 Calories; 2g Fat (satfat 0.5g); 2g Protein; 9g Carbohydrate; 0mg Cholesterol; 105mg Sodium

Raw Apple Cookies

1/2   **cup canola oil**
1/2   **cup brown sugar**
1/4   **cup fructose**
2   **cups unbleached flour**
1/2   **teaspoon salt**
1   **teaspoon vanilla**
1 1/2 cups apple, grated
            COATING
2   **tablespoons fructose**
1   **teaspoon cinnamon**
1   **teaspoon nutmeg**

Combine all ingredients in bowl, working with hands until stiff dough forms. Make into small balls. Roll balls in 2 tablespoons of fructose, 1 teaspoon cinnamon, 1-teaspoon nutmeg. Flatten with fork. Bake at 350 degrees for 15 minutes. *Yield: 3 dozen cookies (serving size 1 cookie)*

Per serving: 65 Calories; 3g Fat (satfat 0.2g); 1g Protein; 8g Carbohydrate; 0mg Cholesterol; 31mg Sodium

Soft Molasses Cookies

*If desired brush with Confectioners' Icing and design
funny faces with raisins and orange slices*

1/2	cup margarine or soy margarine
1/3	cup brown sugar
1/2	cup hot water
1	tablespoon vinegar
1/2	cup molasses
2	egg whites or 1 flax seed egg
2 1/2	cups whole wheat flour *or* unbleached flour
1/2	teaspoon salt
1/4	teaspoon baking soda
1	teaspoon baking powder
1/2	teaspoon ginger
1/2	teaspoon cloves
1	teaspoon cinnamon
1/2	cup raisins

Cream margarine with sugar. In a seperate bowl add hot water and vinegar to the molasses. Combine with margarine and sugar. Add beaten egg. Sift dry ingredients and add. If desired, chop or grind raisins fine and add. Drop dough from teaspoon onto a greased cookie sheet. Bake in a moderate 350°F oven for 15 minutes.

Yield: 7 to 8 dozen cookies (serving size 1 cookie)

🍎🍎🍎🍎🍎

Per serving: 29 Calories; less than one gram Fat (satfat 0.2g); 1g Protein; 5g Carbohydrate; 0mg Cholesterol; 33mg Sodium

Angel Gingerbread

2 1/2	cups unbleached flour
1/2	teaspoon salt
1	teaspoon baking soda
1	teaspoon ginger
1/4	teaspoon cinnamon
1/4	teaspoon nutmeg
1/4	teaspoon allspice
1/2	cup brown sugar
1/2	cup applesauce, unsweetened
2	egg whites + 1 egg *or* 2 flax seed eggs
1/2	cup molasses
1	cup hot water

Sift dry ingredients into a large mixing bowl. Add shortening, eggs, and molasses. With mixer at medium speed, beat 2 minutes. Or beat with spoon 300 strokes. Add hot water and mix well. Pour batter into well-greased 13x9x2-inch pan. Bake 35-40 minutes at 350. Spread Carmel Icing (page 184) over cake in pan. 40 minutes in Bundt pan.

Yield: 24 servings (serving size 1 piece)

Per serving: 84 Calories; less than one gram Fat (satfat 1g); 2g Protein; 18g Carbohydrate; 8mg Cholesterol; 108mg Sodium

Caramel Icing

1/4	cup margarine
1	cup brown sugar
1/4	cup evaporated skim milk *or* soy milk

Melt margarine in saucepan. Add sugar and milk. Stir over medium heat until sugar is dissolved. Bring to a rolling boil (turn heat to high), and then boil 1 minute. Remove from heat and beat immediately. When mixture begins to lose its gloss, spread quickly over cake in pan, while hot. Cool before cutting.

Yield: Will cover (1) 13x9-inch cake

Per serving: 62 Calories; 2g Fat (satfat 0.4); 0g Protein; 11g Carbohydrate; 0mg Cholesterol; 38mg Sodium

Apple Pudding Cake

1	cup brown sugar
4	egg whites + 1 egg or 4 flax seed eggs
1	teaspoon nutmeg
4	large apples, grated
2	teaspoons baking soda
1/2	cup apple juice, frozen concentrate
2	teaspoons cinnamon
1/4	teaspoon salt
2	cups unbleached flour
1	cup walnuts, chopped
2	tablespoons butter

Cream together eggs, sugar, apple juice concentrate and butter. Add remaining ingredients and mix well. Pour into a greased and floured 9 x 13-inch sheet cake pan. Bake at 350° for 40-45 minutes. Serve hot with Nutmeg sauce.
Yield: 24 servings (serving size 1 piece)

🍎🍎🍎🍎🍎

Per serving: 105 Calories; 2g Fat (satfat 0.7); 2g Protein; 20g Carbohydrate; 10mg Cholesterol; 152mg Sodium

Nutmeg Sauce

2	tablespoons cornstarch
1	cup brown sugar
2	cups boiling water
4	tablespoons margarine
2	teaspoons nutmeg *or* vanilla

Mix cornstarch and sugar together and gradually stir in the boiling water. Boil one minute, stirring constantly, then add margarine and nutmeg.
Yield: 2 cups

🍎🍎🍎🍎🍎

Per serving: 114 Calories; 4g Fat (satfat 0.9); 0g Protein; 20g Carbohydrate; 0mg Cholesterol; 59mg Sodium

Banana Cake
Makes a great snack type cake

1/4	cup honey
1	cup apple juice, frozen concentrate
3/4	teaspoon salt
1/2	cup buttermilk *or* soy milk + lemon
1	teaspoon vanilla
2	eggs or 4 tablespoons tofu
1	teaspoon baking soda
1 1/2	cups bananas, mashed
3	cups unbleached flour
1/2	cup canola oil
1	cup coconut
1/2	cup walnuts, toasted and chopped

Cream together sugar, buttermilk, eggs, and bananas. Add remaining ingredients and pour into a 9x13-inch pan. Bake at 350 for 1 hour and 10 minutes. Makes a lot.
Yield: 24 servings*(serving size 1 piece)*

🍎🍎🍎🍎🍎

Per serving: 119 Calories; 3.9g Fat (satfat 1.2g); 2.6g Protein; 22g Carbohydrate; 15mg Cholesterol; 166mg Sodium

Carrot Cake

As compared to regular carrot cake there is no added fats. This cake gets its' moistness from pureed apricots.

1	cup fructose or Natural sugar
3/4	cup apricots, canned, pureed
2	teaspoons baking soda
1 1/2	teaspoons baking powder
2	cups unbleached flour
1/2	cup pecans, toasted and chopped
2	eggs + 3 egg whites or 5 flax seed eggs
2 1/2	teaspoons cinnamon
1	teaspoon salt
2	teaspoons vanilla
1/2	cup crushed pineapple, drained
3	cups carrots, shredded

Cream sugar and apricots together. Add eggs. Combine soda, baking powder, flour, cinnamon, salt, vanilla. Mix well. Add drained pineapple and shredded carrots. Mix well and pour into (3) 9-inch cake pans. Bake at 325° F for 30 minutes or until done. Let cool slightly before removing from pan. Frost with Smooth and Creamy Frosting (page 186) using cheesecake instant pudding for pudding flavor.
Yield: 16-24 servings

Per serving: 132 Calories; 2g Fat (satfat 0.3g); 3g Protein; 26g Carbohydrate; 23mg Cholesterol; 351mg Sodium

Smooth'n Creamy Frosting

The skies the limit on the flavor of frosting with this recipe. Just imagine a light cream cheese frosting using cheesecake pudding. Similar to whipped cream frostings from the bakery, but without all the fat. A real winner!

3	ounces fat-free pudding mix, any flavor
1/4	cup confectioner's sugar
1	cup skim milk *or* soy milk
8	ounces whipped topping, fat free

Combine pudding mix, sugar and milk in small bowl. Beat slowly with rotary beater or at lowest speed of an electric mixer until well-blended, about 1 minute. Fold in whipped topping. Spread on cake at once.
Yield: about 4 cups or enough for two 9-inch layers
Note: Frosted cake should be refrigerated. For a firmer frosting, let mixture stand 5 minutes before folding in whipped topping.

Per serving: 15 Calories; less than one gram Fat (satfat 0g); 0g Protein; 3g Carbohydrate; 0mg Cholesterol; 57mg Sodium

Chocolate-Velvet Cake

6	ounces chocolate chips
2 1/4	cups unbleached flour, sifted
1	teaspoon baking soda
3/4	teaspoon salt
1 1/4	cups honey
3/4	cup prune puree
1	teaspoon vanilla
1	egg + 3 egg white or 1/3 cup tofu

Combine chocolate or carob morsels and 1/4 cup water in saucepan. Stir over low heat until melted and smooth. Remove from heat. Sift flour, soda, and salt together; set aside. Combine sugar, butter and vanilla in bowl; beat until well blended. Add eggs one at a time, beating after each addition. Blend in melted chocolate mixture. Stir in flour mixture alternately with 1-cup water. Pour into 2 greased and floured 9-inch layer pans. Bake at 375 for 30-35 minutes. Cool, and fill layers and cover top with Vanilla Cream Filling or frost with Cocoa White Mountain Frosting.

Yield: 18 servings

🍎🍎🍎🍎🍎

Per serving: 190 Calories; 3g Fat (satfat 1.8g); 3g Protein; 37g Carbohydrate; 10mg Cholesterol; 173mg Sodium

Vanilla Cream Filling

1	cup fructose *or* Natural sugar
3	tablespoons unbleached flour
1/8	teaspoon salt
1 1/2	cups skim milk or soy milk
2	eggs, beaten *or* 2 unflavored gelatin eggs
1/2	teaspoon vanilla

In top of double boiler, mix 1/2-cup sugar, the flour and salt. Add 1/2-cup milk; stir until smooth. Pour in remaining 1-cup milk and cook over boiling water for 10 minutes or until thick and smooth; stirring constantly, mix remaining 1/4-cup sugar and the eggs. Add to hot mixture slowly, stirring constantly. Put back in double boiler and cook 5 minutes or until thick. Let cool then add the vanilla. *Yield: Makes enough to fill four 8-inch or three 9-inch layers.*

🍎🍎🍎🍎🍎

Per serving: 57 Calories; 1g Fat (satfat 0.2g); 2g Protein; 12g Carbohydrate; 23mg Cholesterol; 36mg Sodium

White Mountain Frosting

1/2	cup fructose
1/4	cup light corn syrup
2	tablespoons water
2	egg whites
1	teaspoon vanilla

Combine fructose, corn syrup and water in small saucepan. Cover; heat to rolling boil over medium heat. Remove cover and boil rapidly, without stirring, to 242° on candy thermometer (or until small amount of mixture spins a 6 to 8-inch thread when dropped from a spoon).

As mixture boils, beat egg whites until stiff peaks form. Pour hot syrup very slowly in a thin stream into the beaten egg whites, beating constantly on medium speed. Beat on high speed until stiff peaks form; add vanilla during last minute of beating.

Yield: fills and frosts two 8 or 9-inch layers or one 13 x 9-inch cake.

Variations on a Theme

- Cocoa Frosting: Sift 1/4-cup cocoa over frosting and gently fold in until blended.
- Lemon Frosting: Substitute 1 tablespoon lemon juice for the vanilla and add 1/4 teaspoon grated lemon peel and 10 drops yellow food color during last minute of beating.
- Pink Mountain Frosting: Substitute maraschino cherry juice for the water.

🍎🍎🍎🍎🍎

Per serving: 35 Calories; 0g Fat (satfat 0); 0g Protein; 9g Carbohydrate; 0mg Cholesterol; 14mg Sodium

Fresh Apple Cake With Cinnamon Butter

2	cups wheat flour
2	teaspoons baking powder
1	teaspoon salt
1/2	teaspoon cinnamon
1/4	teaspoon nutmeg
1/2	cup applesauce
3/4	cup honey
2	eggs *or* 2 flax seed eggs
1 1/2	cups apple, grated
1/2	cup pecans, toasted and chopped

Sift together flour, baking powder, salt, cinnamon and nutmeg. Cream butter and honey together until light and fluffy. Beat in eggs, one at a time, beating hard after each addition. Stir in dry ingredients and apple, half at a time. Fold in pecans. Grease and flour a 9 by 5 by 3-inch loaf pan. Pour batter into prepared pan and bake in a 350° oven for one hour or until cake is done. Cool in pan for 10 minutes. Turn out onto a wire rack to cook completely before slicing. Serve with Cinnamon butter.
Yield: 16 servings

CINNAMON BUTTER: Cream 3 tablespoons butter with 1/2 cup honey and 1/4 teaspoon of cinnamon. Whip until creamy. Chill before serving.

🍎🍎🍎🍎🍎

Per serving: 131 Calories; 2g Fat (satfat 0.3g); 3g Protein; 28g Carbohydrate; 23mg Cholesterol; 187mg Sodium

German Chocolate Cake

1/2	cup boiling water
4	ounces German chocolate squares
3/4	cup pear puree (6oz jar baby food) or canola oil
1/4	cup margarine, softened
1 1/2	cups fructose
2	flax seed eggs *or* 2 egg yolks
1	teaspoon vanilla
2 1/2	cups unbleached flour
1 1/2	teaspoons baking soda
1/4	teaspoon salt
1	cup buttermilk *or* soy milk + lemon
4	egg whites, stiffly beaten *or* 4 unflavored gelatin eggs

Heat oven to 350°F. Grease 3 round layer pans. Line bottoms of pans with waxed paper. In small bowl, pour boiling water over chocolate, stirring until chocolate is melted; set aside to cool.

In large mixer bowl, cream pears, margarine and fructose until smooth. Beat in flaxseed egg. On low speed, blend in chocolate and vanilla. Mix in flour, baking soda and salt alternately with buttermilk, beating after each addition until batter is smooth. Fold in egg whites. Divide batter among pans.

Bake 25 to 30 minutes or until top springs back when touched lightly with finger. Cool. Fill layers and frost top of cake with Coconut-Pecan Frosting. *Yield: 16-24 servings*

🍎🍎🍎🍎🍎

Per serving: 200 Calories; 5g Fat (satfat 0.6g); 4g Protein; 36g Carbohydrate; 1mg Cholesterol; 178 mg Sodium

Coconut-Pecan Frosting

1 1/2	cups evaporated skim milk
3/4	cup natural sugar or fructose
2	egg yolks
1	tablespoon cornstarch *or* arrowroot
3	tablespoons Molly McButter®
1	teaspoon vanilla
1 1/3	cups coconut flakes
3/4	cup pecans, toasted and chopped

Combine evaporated milk, sugar, egg yolks, cornstarch, Molly McButter, water and vanilla in small saucepan. Cook and stir over medium heat until thick, about 12 minutes. Stir in coconut and pecans. Beat until thick enough to spread. *Yield: 2 1/2 cups.*

🍎🍎🍎🍎🍎

Per serving: 69 Calories; 3g Fat (satfat 1.4); 2g Protein; 9g Carbohydrate; 18mg Cholesterol; 99mg Sodium

Oatmeal Cake

1	cup oats, rolled (cooked)
1 1/2	cups boiling water
3/4	cup brown sugar
2/3	cup apple juice, frozen concentrate
1	egg or 1 flax seed egg
1	teaspoon cinnamon
2	tablespoons margarine or soy margarine
1 1/2	cups unbleached flour
2	teaspoons baking powder
1/4	teaspoon salt

In a bowl put oats. Pour boiling water over oats and let stand while preparing cake batter. To prepare batter cream together sugar, apple juice concentrate, cinnamon and margarine. Add oatmeal and mix well. Blend in flour, baking powder, egg and salt, mix till smooth. Pour into a floured and greased 9x13-inch pan. Bake at 350°F for 35 minutes. Frost with Coconut-Pecan Icing found on page 185 or Brown Sugar Frosting found below. ..
Yield: 24 servings

🍎🍎🍎🍎🍎🍎

Per serving: 73 Calories; 1g Fat (satfat 0.2); 1g Protein; 15g Carbohydrate; 8mg Cholesterol; 67mg Sodium

Brown Sugar Frosting

1/2	cup brown sugar
1/4	cup dark corn syrup
2	tablespoons water
2	egg whites
1/2	teaspoon vanilla

Combine brown sugar, corn syrup and water in small saucepan. Cover; heat to rolling boil over medium heat. Remove cover and boil rapidly, without stirring, to 242° on candy thermometer (or until small amount of mixture spins a 6 to 8-inch thread when dropped from a spoon).

As mixture boils, beat egg whites until stiff peaks form. Pour hot syrup very slowly in a thin stream into the beaten egg whites, beating constantly on medium speed. Beat on high speed until stiff peaks form; add vanilla during last minute of beating.
Yield: fills and frosts two 8 or 9-inch layers or one 13 x 9-inch cake.

🍎🍎🍎🍎🍎🍎

Per serving: 35 Calories; 0g Fat (satfat 0); 0g Protein; 9g Carbohydrate; 0mg Cholesterol; 14mg Sodium

For Health's Sake

Pinto Bean Cake

Beans never tasted so Good!

Sweet Treats

1	cup apple juice frozen concentrate, thawed
1/4	cup brown sugar
1 1/2	cups pinto beans, mashed
2	flax seed eggs *or* 2 egg whites + 1 egg
3/4	cup apple, grated
1	teaspoon lemon juice
2	cups unbleached flour
2	teaspoons baking powder
1/2	teaspoon salt
1/2	teaspoon nutmeg
1/2	teaspoon cinnamon
1/4	cup raisins

Combine apple juice concentrate and beans. Beat in eggs, apples, and lemon juice. Add dry ingredients and beat well. Add raisins. Pour into a greased and floured 9x13-inch-baking pan. Bake at 350°F for 40 to 50 minutes. Frost with Smooth'n Creamy Frosting (use lemon pudding for the pudding flavor) on page 186.

Yield: 24 servings

Variation on a Theme

Leave out the nutmeg and replace raisins with 1-cup miniature chocolate chips and frost with Magic Chocolate Frosting..

🍎🍎🍎🍎🍎🍎

Per serving: 111 Calories; less than one gram Fat (satfat 0.1g); 4g Protein; 24g Carbohydrate; 0mg Cholesterol; 50mg Sodium

Magic Chocolate Frosting

1	can sweetened condensed milk, fat free
1	tablespoon water
	dash salt
2	squares unsweetened baking chocolate squares
1/2	teaspoon vanilla

Combine in top of double boiler sweetened condensed milk, water, salt and chocolate. Cook over boiling water until thick stirring constantly until thick. Remove from the heat and cool. Stir in vanilla and then spread on cooled cake. Has the taste of thick fudge. *Yield: 1 1/2 cups*

🍎🍎🍎🍎🍎🍎

Per serving: 26 Calories; 2g Fat (satfat 1.2g); 1g Protein; 3g Carbohydrate; 0mg Cholesterol; 3mg Sodium

Pumpkin Nut Cake

3	cups wheat flour *or* unbleached flour
2	tablespoons baking powder
1/4	teaspoon salt
2	eggs + 4 egg whites or 5 flax seed eggs
2	cups pumpkin
1 1/2	teaspoons baking soda
1	tablespoon cinnamon
1	cup molasses
1	cup applesauce
1	cup walnuts, toasted and chopped

Put honey or molasses, eggs, pumpkin and oil in bowl and mix well. Then add flour, baking powder, salt, soda, cinnamon and mix well. After everything is mixed well, fold in the nuts. Pour cake mix into a sheet cake pan or loaf pans. Bake at 350° F for 55 minutes. Frost this cake with Caramel Icing on page 188 or Brown Sugar Frosting found on page 186. .
Yield: 24 servings

🍎🍎🍎🍎🍎

Per serving: 114 Calories; 1g Fat (satfat 0.2g); 3g Protein; 24g Carbohydrate; 15mg Cholesterol; 212mg Sodium

Rhubarb Cake

1	cup brown sugar
1/2	cup margarine or soy margarine
2	egg whites *or* 1 flax seed eggs
1	cup plain lowfat yogurt
2	cups unbleached flour
1 1/2	teaspoons baking soda
1 1/2	teaspoons vanilla
1 1/2	cups rhubarb cut into small pieces
1/2	cup fructose
1	tablespoon cinnamon

Cream brown sugar and margarine. Add egg. Combine flour and baking soda. Add to creamed mixture alternate with yogurt. Add vanilla and rhubarb. Pour into greased and floured 13x9x2-inch pan. Combine fructose and cinnamon. Sprinkle over batter. Bake at 350° for 50 minutes.
Yield: 24 servings

🍎🍎🍎🍎🍎

Per serving: 101 Calories; 2.6g Fat (satfat 0.6g); 2g Protein; 17g Carbohydrate; 1mg Cholesterol; 126mg Sodium

Fresh Strawberry Pie

*A refreshing light pie. Nobody believes me when I tell them
that it is low-fat and low sugar.*

3   ounces strawberry gelatin powder
1 2/3 cups boiling water
1   tablespoon fructose
1 1/2 cups fresh strawberries, sliced
1   9-inch graham cracker crust, reduced fat non-dairy whipped
       topping or sweetened soy yogurt

Dissolve gelatin and fructose in boiling water. Chill gelatin until thickened. Stir
in strawberries. Pour into pie shell and return to the refrigerator until firm, at
least 3 hours. Serve with a dollop of whipped topping or sweetened yogurt.
Garnish with fresh berries.
Yield: 1 pie or 8 slices

Variations on a Theme

When the summer months bring on a variety of fresh fruit I make this pie
repeatedly. One of my husband's favorite combinations is strawberries and
raspberries, the more the merrier. Be creative. This is a basic recipe, so try
different flavors of gelatin with different fruit like; fresh apricots in apricot gelatin
or fresh blueberries in a berry flavored gelatin. The combinations are endless
… so have fun.

🍎🍎🍎🍎🍎

Per serving: 54 Calories; less than one gram Fat (satfat 0g); 1g Protein; 13g
Carbohydrate; 0mg Cholesterol; 30mg Sodium

Sweet Treats

German Chocolate Pie

A very satisfying chocolate fix. A real crowd pleaser.

1/2	pound marshmallows (30-32 large)
1/8	teaspoon salt
1	cup skim milk or almond milk
1	teaspoon vanilla
2	cups fat-free whipped topping
1/4	cup coconut
1/2	cup chocolate chips
1/4	cup pecans, toasted and chopped
1	No Fail Pie Crust, baked

Add marshmallows, chocolate, and milk over double boiler until melted. Cool and stir in salt and vanilla, fold in whipped cream, coconut, and nuts. Pour into shell and chill. (Chocolate goes lumpy and uneven if it is not cooled). Garnish with whipped cream and shaved chocolate.
Yield: 1 pie or 8 slices

🍎🍎🍎🍎🍎

Per serving: 214 Calories; 6g Fat (satfat 2.4g); 2g Protein; 39g Carbohydrate; 1mg Cholesterol; 97mg Sodium

Honey Pumpkin Pie

No Thanksgiving celebration is complete without
pumpkin pie and this one is very low in fat too!

16	ounces pumpkin, canned
3/4	cup honey
1	teaspoon cinnamon
1/2	teaspoon salt
1/2	teaspoon ginger
1/4	teaspoon nutmeg
1/2	teaspoon cloves
1/2	teaspoon allspice
1	large egg + 3 egg whites or 1/3 cup tofu
2/3	cup evaporated skim milk or almond milk
2	tablespoons flour
1	9 inch No Fail Pie Crust

In a larger mixing bowl, stir together pumpkin, honey, cinnamon, salt, ginger, nutmeg, allspice and cloves. Add eggs. Beat eggs into pumpkin mixture with a fork. Stir in cream, and flour; mix well. Prepare piecrust for filling. Bake in 375° oven for 55 to 60 minutes or till a knife inserted in center comes out clean. Serve hot or cold with fresh whipped topping.
Yield: 1 pie or 8 slices

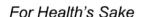

Per serving: 171 Calories; 2g Fat (satfat 0.4g); 5g Protein; 37g Carbohydrate; 23mg Cholesterol; 202mg Sodium

Nectarine and Peach Pie
Give me a spoon and let me indulge. Excellent Pie!
Fran, kitchen tester

1	cup nectarines, peeled and sliced
3	cups peaches, peeled and sliced
1/2	cup fructose or natural sugar
1/4	teaspoon salt
2 1/2	tablespoons unbleached flour or tapioca
1	9 inch No Fail Pie Crust
	CRUMBS
5	tablespoons margarine, melted
1/2	cup unbleached flour
1	teaspoon cinnamon
1/2	cup brown sugar

Peel and slice peaches and nectarines. In a large bowl mix gently together fruit, fructose, salt and flour. Let blend for 5 minutes before spooning into pie shell.

To make crumbs melt margarine in bowl. Add flour, cinnamon and brown sugar. Mix together until crumbly. Cover top of pie with crumbs. Bake at 425°F for 45 -50 minutes. *Yield: 1 9-inch pie or 8 servings*

Variation on a Theme
When this pie was tested at the tasting party lots of people told me to forget the piecrust and just serve it as a crisp. If you do this you will save yourself some fat calories (0.9).

Personal Note: This recipe is based on an old Amish recipe for peach pie. But when I had more nectarines and peaches than I could eat I combined them for this delicious treat.

🍎🍎🍎🍎🍎

Per serving: 195 Calories; 5g Fat (satfat 1.0g); 2g Protein; 35g Carbohydrate; 0mg Cholesterol; 147mg Sodium

No Fail Pie Crust

A flaky piecrust, that is easy to make and low in saturated fat. Compare to a regular piecrust with 130 calories and 8 grams of fat per serving (satfat 5g).

2	cups unbleached flour
1/2	teaspoon salt
1/2	cup canola oil or corn oil
1/4	cup skim milk or soy milk, cold

Mix together sifted flour and salt. Add oil and milk. Stir until mixed well. Divide into two balls. Roll between sheets of waxed paper.
Yield: 2 piecrusts or one double crust

Personal Note: The secret to a tender, flaky piecrust is to handle it as little as possible when mixing and rolling.

Per serving: 118 Calories; 7g Fat (satfat 0.5); 2g Protein; 12g Carbohydrate; 0mg Cholesterol; 69mg Sodium

Apple Macaroon

4	medium apples
1/2	cup brown sugar
1/2	teaspoon cinnamon
1/2	cup coconut
1/3	cup pecans, toasted and chopped
3	tablespoons canola oil
1/4	cup plain lowfat yogurt or soy yogurt
1/3	cup fructose
3/4	cup unbleached flour
2	egg whites, well-beaten or unflavored gelatin eggs
1/2	teaspoon vanilla

Mix brown sugar, cinnamon, nuts and coconut together. In a 10" pie pan sprinkle sugar mixture. To make batter cream together fructose, egg whites, yogurt and oil. Stir in flour and vanilla gently. Place sliced apples on top of sugar mixture, and then pour batter over apples. Bake at 375° for 35 minutes.
Yield: 10-12 servings

Per serving: 174 Calories; 6g Fat (satfat 1.1); 2g Protein; 28g Carbohydrate; 0mg Cholesterol; 19mg Sodium

Sweet Treats

Boston Cream Pie

2	cups unbleached flour
2 1/2	teaspoons baking powder
1/2	teaspoon salt
1	cup apple juice, frozen concentrate, thawed
1	teaspoon vanilla
1/4	teaspoon almond extract
1	egg *or* 2 tablespoons tofu

CUSTARD CREAM FILLING

1	cup skim milk or almond milk
1/2	cup fructose or natural sugar
3	tablespoons cornstarch *or* arrowroot
	dash salt
2	eggs or 4 tablespoons tofu
1	tablespoon butter
1	teaspoon vanilla

Sift together dry ingredients into mixing bowl. Add shortening, milk, vanilla and almond extract. Beat 2 minutes, using medium speed on electric mixer or 300 strokes by hand. Add egg; beat 2 minutes more. Pour into two greased 8" or 9" round layer cake pans. Bake in moderate oven 350, for 25 to 30 minutes. Cool on racks. Use one layer to make Boston Cream Pie; freeze the other for later use. Split cooled cake layer in crosswise halves. Spread Custard Cream Filling over lower half. If desire spread Chocolate icing over the outside and you have Chocolate Cream Pie.

To make the filling add milk gradually to mixture of 1/2-cup fructose, cornstarch and salt. Cook slowly, stirring constantly, until mixture thickens, about 10 to 15 minutes. Add about 1/2 cup hot mixture to the 2 eggs and blend; carefully combine both mixtures and cook about 3 minutes, stirring constantly. Remove from heat; blend in 1-tablespoon butter and 1-teaspoon vanilla.
Yield: 8 -10 pieces

Variations on a Theme
For a scrumptious cake, split both layers and add 1 cup shredded coconut and 1/2 cup chopped nuts to custard. Then frost with chocolate frosting. Or for Banana custard cream filling spread cake with filling, then cover filling with banana slices.

🍎🍎🍎🍎🍎

Per serving: 269 Calories; 4g Fat (satfat 1.5); 6g Protein; 53g Carbohydrate; 72mg Cholesterol; 308mg Sodium

Chocolate Pudding Desert

1	cup unbleached flour
1/2	cup margarine, melted
1/2	cup walnuts, toasted and chopped
8	ounces cream cheese, fat free
16	ounces whipped topping, fat free
1	cup powdered sugar
1	package chocolate fat-free pudding mix
1	package white chocolate or cheesecake fat-free pudding mix
3	cups skim milk, or oat milk
	chocolate, grated

Preheat oven to 350°. Melt margarine. Pour graham cracker crumbs into bottom of a 9x13 inch pan, pour margarine over crumbs and mix well. Press crumbs into bottom of pan. Set in refrigerator to set while you mix remaining ingredients. Mix together cream cheese, 2 1/2 cups cool whip and powdered sugar until smooth. Spread cream cheese mix over crust. Mix milk and both packages of pudding together until smooth. Spread pudding mix over cream cheese mix. For final layer spread remaining whipped topping over pudding and sprinkle with grated chocolate. Refrigerate for 1-2 hours till set.

🍎🍎🍎🍎🍎

Per serving: 90 Calories; 3g Fat (satfat 0.6); 3g Protein; 12g Carbohydrate; 2mg Cholesterol; 128mg Sodium

Flan - French Style

2	eggs *or* 1/4 cup tofu
1 1/4	cups skim milk *or* soy milk
1	tablespoon honey
1	teaspoon vanilla
	nutmeg

Beat eggs. Add milk, honey and vanilla; blend well. Pour into four 6-ounce custard cups. Sprinkle with nutmeg. Place in baking pan with deep sides. Add hot water to 1/2-inch depth. Bake at 350° about 40 minutes or until knife inserted in center comes out clean.
Yield: 4 6-ounce custards

Variation on a Theme
Just for fun try different flavorings, like mint, strawberry, almond, etc. If you want, add a few drops of food coloring to it to match the taste.

🍎🍎🍎🍎🍎

Per serving: 76 Calories; 2g Fat (satfat 0.8); 5g Protein; 8g Carbohydrate; 92mg Cholesterol; 66mg Sodium

Raisin Apple Betty

3	cups soft bread crumbs
1/2	cup raisins, seedless
1	apple diced
3	tablespoons margarine or soy margarine
1/2	cup brown sugar, packed
1/4	cup water
1/4	teaspoon cinnamon

Pare apple, core and cut into thin slices. Place 1 cup bread crumbs in baking pan, add half the apple, raisins, and sugar. Dot with 1-tablespoon butter. Add another cup crumbs, remaining apple, raisins, sugar and dot with butter. Cover with remaining crumbs. Add remaining butter and sprinkle with cinnamon. Add water. Cover dish and bake about 1 hour at 350. Serve warm or cold with cream.
Yield: 12 servings

🍎🍎🍎🍎🍎🍎

Per serving: 175 Calories; 4g Fat (satfat 0.8); 3g Protein; 32g Carbohydrate; 0mg Cholesterol; 217mg Sodium

Simple Country Cheese Cake

3	cups cottage cheese, lowfat *or* silken tofu
5	eggs, slightly beaten or 5 flax seed eggs
1/4	teaspoon salt
1	teaspoon vanilla
1/4	teaspoon almond extract
1/2	cup fructose or natural sugar
3/4	cup flour
1 1/2	cups evaporated skim milk or soy milk
	jam or fresh fruit

Press cottage cheese through sieve (or blend with 1 cup of milk in blender until smooth). Add eggs, salt, vanilla and almond extract to cheese; blend thoroughly. Combine sugars and flour; slowly blend into cheese mixture. Add milk. Pour into buttered 9" square pan. Set dish in pan of water. Bake in moderate oven 350° for 1 hour or until knife inserted comes out clean. Cool. Serve with jam or fruit and whipped topping.
Yield: 12 servings

🍎🍎🍎🍎🍎🍎

Per serving: 145 Calories; 2g Fat (satfat 1.0); 12g Protein; 18g Carbohydrate; 79mg Cholesterol; 333mg Sodium

Swiss Strawberry Rice

1	cup rice
3	cups skim milk *or* almond milk
1/4	cup fructose
1/2	teaspoon salt
2	eggs beaten or 4 tablespoons tofu
1 1/2	cups whipped topping, fat free
1	teaspoon almond extract
10	ounces frozen strawberries, sliced

Cook rice and milk together in top of double boiler until tender, stirring occasionally, about 1 hour. Add sugar and salt. Add a little hot mixture gradually to beaten eggs. Stir eggs into remaining mixture. Blend well; cook 1 minute and cool. Fold whipped topping and almond extract into rice. Chill. Serve with partly thawed strawberries.
Yield: 8 servings

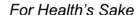

Per serving: 201 Calories; 1g Fat (satfat 0.5); 6g Protein; 40g Carbohydrate; 47mg Cholesterol; 211mg Sodium

Almond Crunch Candy

1/3	cup margarine or butter
1/4	cup honey
3/4	cup almonds, slivered

Butter 8x8-inch shallow pan. Melt margarine in heavy frying pan; stir in honey. Add almonds. Cook over medium heat, stirring constantly until mix turns golden brown, about 7 minutes. Spread mix into prepared pan; work quickly, while still hot. With buttered sharp knife cut into squares immediately. Cool. Chill in refrigerator and store in covered container.
Yield: 36 pieces

Per serving: 24 Calories; 2g Fat (satfat 0.3g); 0g Protein; 2g Carbohydrate; 0mg Cholesterol; 15mg Sodium

Cashew Brittle

3/4	cup honey
1/4	cup water
1	cup raw cashews
1	tablespoon margarine
1/2	teaspoon vanilla
1	teaspoon baking soda

In an iron skillet, boil honey and water until it forms a soft ball when dropped into cold water or reaches 234° F. Add nuts and continue to boil until golden brown, about 10 to 12 minutes, stirring continuously. Remove from heat and add butter, vanilla, and soda. Mix well, then pour onto a greased cookie sheet. When cool, break into pieces.

Yield: 36 pieces or about 1 pound.

🍎🍎🍎🍎🍎

Per serving: 44 Calories; 2g Fat (satfat 0.4g); 1g Protein; 7g Carbohydrate; 0mg Cholesterol; 39mg Sodium

Creme Caramels

1 1/3	cups honey
1/2	cup margarine or butter
2	cups evaporated skim milk

Combine honey, margarine and 1 cup of milk in saucepan. Bring to boil, stirring frequently. Cook until mixture begins to darken and thicken. Add remaining milk and continue to cook until mixture forms a fairly firm ball when dropped into cold water or reaches 244° F. Pour into buttered 8x8-inch pan. When cool, cut into 1-inch squares and wrap individually.

Yield: 64 1-inch pieces

Variations on a Theme
Add 1/2 cup toasted nuts 5 minutes before finished cooking. When cool, cut into squares and dip into a chocolate coating mix. Great for holiday gift giving.

🍎🍎🍎🍎🍎

Per serving: 36 Calories;less than 1 gram of Fat (satfat 0.2g), 0.6g Protein; 6.7g Carbohydrate; 0mg Cholesterol; 22mg Sodium

Fruit-Jelly Candies

1   cup orange juice *or* favorite juice
1/2   cup pectin liquid
1/2   cup fructose or natural sugar
1/2   cup honey

Mix juice and pectin together in saucepan. Add sugar and honey, stirring. Heat juice mixture to boiling, stirring. Cook until syrup drops in a sheet from spoon. Remove from heat. Pour syrup to 3/4-inch depth in shallow pan. Set aside overnight. Cut fruit jelly into squares. Place on waxed paper and set aside 24 hours.

Yield: 24 squares

Variations on a Theme
1/2 cup chopped nuts. Add nuts after removing from heat.
1 cup chopped dried fruit. Add fruit after removing from heat.
Peppermint flavoring and green food coloring. Add after removing from heat.

Per serving: 54 Calories; 0g Fat (satfat 0g); 0.1g Protein; 15g Carbohydrate; 0mg Cholesterol; 11mg Sodium

Maple-Glazed Nuts

1/2   cup maple syrup
1   teaspoon cinnamon
1   tablespoon margarine
1/4   teaspoon salt
1 1/2   teaspoons vanilla
2   cups walnuts

In an iron skillet stir together syrup, cinnamon, butter and salt. Cook and stir over medium heat until mixture becomes brown and starts to thicken. Add vanilla, then nuts and toss until nuts are all covered evenly with glaze. Cool on wax paper.
Yield about 2 cups.

Per serving: 36 Calories; 2g Fat (satfat 0.2g); 1g Protein; 5g Carbohydrate; 0mg Cholesterol; 27mg Sodium

Molasses Candy

1   **teaspoon margarine**
1   **cup dark molasses**
1   **tablespoon water**
1/4 **cup brown sugar**
1/4 **teaspoon baking soda**

Melt the butter in a heavy skillet; add molasses, water and sugar, and stir until sugar is dissolved. Stir occasionally until nearly done, and then constantly. Boil until the spoon leaves a track in the bottom of pan while stirring, to hard-ball stage, 255° F. Stir well, add the soda, stir thoroughly, and pour in a very well greased pan. When cool enough to handle, pull until light colored and porous. Work candy with fingertips and thumbs; do not squeeze in the hands. When it begins to harden, stretch to the desire thickness, cut in small pieces with large shears. Cool on buttered plate.
Yield: 24 pieces

🍎🍎🍎🍎🍎

Per serving: 43 Calories; less than one gram Fat (satfat 0g); 0g Protein; 11g Carbohydrate; 0mg Cholesterol; 15mg Sodium

Penuche

2   **cups brown sugar**
3/4 **cup milk, skim or rice milk**
2   **tablespoons margarine**
1   **teaspoon vanilla**
2   **cups walnuts, chopped**

Boil sugar and milk to the soft-ball stage 236° F. Remove from heat; add butter, nuts and flavoring. Cool to lukewarm. Beat until creamy and thickened; press into a greased square pan, and when firm, cut into squares.
Yield: 64 1-inch squares

🍎🍎🍎🍎🍎

Per serving: 26 Calories; less than 1 gram of Fat; (satfat 0.1g); 0.3g Protein; 4.7g Carbohydrate; 0mg Cholesterol; 6mg Sodium

Quick Fudge

1	package chocolate chips
1	cup sweetened condensed milk, fat free
1	teaspoon vanilla
2/3	cup walnuts, toasted and chopped

Heat chips and condensed milk in saucepan over low heat, stirring until chocolate is melted. Remove from heat; blend in vanilla. Spread in buttered 8-inch square pan. Chill until firm, at least 4 hours. Cut into 1-inch squares.
Yield: 64 1-inch squares

🍎🍎🍎🍎🍎🍎

Per serving: 28 Calories; 1g Fat (satfat 0.5g); 0.6g Protein; 4.7g Carbohydrate; 0mg Cholesterol; 5mg Sodium

Spanish Sweets

1/4	pound candied cherries, chopped
1/4	pound seedless raisins, chopped
1/4	pound figs, chopped
1/4	pound dates, pitted and chopped
1/4	pound almonds, chopped
1/2	pound walnuts, chopped
1/4	pound pecans, chopped

Mix all together and grind fine or chop. Sprinkle board with pulverized or powdered sugar, toss on the mixture, and knead well. Roll out to about 1/2 thick. Cut into small squares. Will keep packed in layers between sheets of waxed paper.
Yield: 2 pounds or about 48 1 -1 1/2 inch squares.

🍎🍎🍎🍎🍎🍎

Per serving: 38 Calories; 2g Fat (satfat 0.2g); 0.7g Protein; 5g Carbohydrate;

0mg Cholesterol; 2mg Sodi

My Good Book List

A World Without Cancer, The Story of Vitamin B-17, G. Edward Griffin, American Media, 1978.

Cooking Without Fat, George Mateljan, Health Valley Foods, 1992, ISBN 0-9633608-0-9

Jane Brody's Good Food Book, Living the High-Carbohydrate Way, Jane Brody, Penguin Books, 1985, ISBN

The King Arthur Flour 200th Anniversary Cookbook, Brinna B. Sands, Countryman Press, 1991.

Grains, Bonnie Tandy Lebland and Joanne Lamb Hayes, Harmony Books, 1995.

Cooking the Whole Foods Way, Christina Pirello, Berkley Publishing, 1997.

366 Simply Delicious Dairy-Free Recipes, Robin Robertson, Penguin Group, 1997.

Cooking with Home Storage, Peggy Layton, 1991, (888) 835-0311.

Eat to Win, The Sports Nutrition Bible, Robert Haas, Signet Books, 1983.

Runner's World Natural Foods Cookbook, Pamela Hannan, Runner's World Books, 1983, ISBN 0-89037-275-6.

Chef Sato's All Natural Desserts, Satoru Sato, One Peaceful World Press, 1998, ISBN 1-882984-32-3.

Get the Fat Out, Victoria Moran, Crown Publishers, 1994, ISBN 0-517-88184-5.

Great Web Sites to Check Out

http://www.5aday.com
http://www.goodstuffonline.com
http://www.oldwayspt.org
http://www.delicious-online.com
http://www.iVillage.com
http://www.intelihealth.com
http://www.soar.Berkeley.EDU/recipes/Healthy.net
http://www.Healthwell.com
http://www.nutritiouslygourmet.com
http://www.nalusda.gov/fnic/dga/dguide95.html
http://www.excite.com/lifestyle/food_and_drink/recipes/health_conscious/
http://www.healthyideas.com
http://www.floridacrystals.com
http://www.wholefoods.com

Bibliography

Chapter 2: Healing the Body and Soul
Go Heavy on the Veggies to Prevent Cancer, The New York Times
　　Syndicate, 1999
Doctorineand Covenants, Section 89:10-16, 1833.

Chapter 3: Wheat and Other Grains of Knowledge
Jane Brody's Good Food Book, Living the High-Carbohydrate Way,
　　Jane Brody, Penguin Books, 1985, p.39-42
The King Arthur Flour 200th Anniversary Cookbook, Brinna B. Sands,
　　Countryman Press, 1991 p.9-11.
Grains, Bonnie Tandy Lebland and Joanne Lamb Hayes, Harmony
　　Books, 1995, p. 5, 9-14

Chapter 4: Fruity and Fresh
*The Power of Eating Right Studies Show Diet High In Fruits & Veg-
　　etables Reduces Health Risk*, press release by Elizabeth Pivonka,
　　Ph.D., RD for Produce for Better Health, www.5aday.com, February
　　9, 1998.
Do Yourself A Flavor, Graham Kerr and Elizabeth Pivonka, A series by
　　the Produce For Better Health Foundation, www.5aday.com, 1999.
Jane Brody's Good Food Book, Living the High-Carbohydrate Way,
　　W.W. Norton & Co., 1985, p. 126-127.

Chapter 5: Veggie Power
Do Yourself A Flavor, Graham Kerr and Elizabeth Pivonka, A series by
　　the Produce For Better Health Foundation, www.5aday.com, 1999.
Jane Brody's Good Food Book, Living the High-Carbohydrate Way,
　　Jane Brody, Penguin Books, 1985.
Vegetables, Elson M. Haas, M.D., www.Healthy.net, 1999

Chapter 6: Bowled Over by Beans
Bean Cuisine, Heather McPherson, Orlando Sentinel, January 1,
　　1998.
Jane Brody's Good Food Book, Living the High-Carbohydrate Way,
　　Jane Brody, Penguin Books, 1985

Chapter 7: Seasonings by Herb
Cooking with Home Storage, Peggy Layton, 1991, (888) 835-0311.

Chapter 8: Mooove Over Dairy
Ten Reasons to Eat Dairy, Sue Gilbert and Fran Clinton, www.iVillage.com, 1999
Better Homes and Gardens, Complete Guide to Food and Cooking, Meredith Corporation, 1991.
Dairy Products, Elson M. Haas, M.D., www.Healthy.net, 1999
Jane Brody's Good Food Book, Living the High Carbohydrate Way, W.W. Norton & Company, 1985.
Cooking the Whole Foods Way, Christina Pirello, Berkley Publishing, 1997.
366 Simply Delicious Dairy-Free Recipes, Robin Robertson, Penguin Group, 1997.

Chapter 9: Getting Off the Fat-Go-Round
Fat Ain't Where It's At, Jean Williams, Deseret News, March 29, 1994.
Cooking Without Fat, George Mateljan, Health Valley Foods, 1992, p. 368
Eat to Win, The Sports Nutrition Bible, Robert Haas, Signet Books, 1983, p. 220-221.
Fat is Not a Four Letter Word, Sue Gilbert, www.iVillage.com , 1999.

Chapter 10: The Truth about Sweeteners
The Sweet Surrender, Steven Pratt, Chicago Tribune, March 28, 1996
Guide to Sweeteners, Ken Babal, C.N., Health Store News, December 1993/January 1994, p. 17

Chapter 11: Oh No I'm Out of ... A Guide to Substitutions
Orlando *Sentinel,* Test kitchen; Cathy Barber, Universal Press Syndicate; *Chicago Tribune* Test kitchen; *Sun-Sentinel*, South Florida
Joy of Cooking (Bobbs-Merrill)
Kitchen Solutions: Substitutions, Basic Formulas and Essential References, Bristol Publishing
Jane Brody's Good Food Book, Living the High Carbohydrate Way (Norton and Co.)
Cooking with Home Storage, Peggy Layton, 1991, (888) 835-0311.

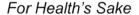
Index

A

Alfredo Sauce 155
Almond Citrus Salad 85
Almond Crunch Candy 197
Amazing Crustless Quiche 138
Ambrosia Platter 86
Angel Gingerbread 178
Appetizer
  Baked Tortilla Chips 55
  Calcutta 56
  Celery Pinwheels 57
  Chi Tan Chuan (Chinese Egg
      Rolls) 56
  Devilish Eggs 57
  Salmon Log 59
  Stuffed Cucumbers 59
Apple-Cinnamon Granola 66
Apple-Peach Granola 67
Applesauce-Spice Cookies 166
Apple Bran Muffins 97
Apple Gratin 117
Apple Macaroon 193
Apple Pudding Cake 179
Apple Salad 84
Ardy's Clam Chowder 77

B

Baby Carrots with Curry Sauce 119
Baked Lentils 139
Baked Tortilla Chips 55
Banana Cake 180
Barbecue Sauce 156
Basic Sugar Cookies 167
Basic White Sauce 155
Bean Sprout Casserole 119
Berry Cream Muffins 98
Beverages
  Cherry/Apple Drink 60
  Citrus Refresher 60
  Fruit Smoothie 61

Good Luck Punch 61
Hot Apple Punch 62
Island Sunset 62
Old Fashioned Lemonade 63
Orange-Apricot Spritzer 63
Plum Refresher 64
Rhubarb Slush 64
Tropical Slush 65
V-7 Juice 65
Very Berry Cooler 66
Bibliography 203
Boston Cream Pie 194
Bowled Over by Beans 33
Breads
  Apple Bran Muffins 97
  French Bread 112
  Golden Raisin Buns 100
  Granny's Whole Wheat Bread
      108
  Herbed Oatmeal Pan Bread 107
  Honey Graham Crackers 101
  Icebox Butterhorns 108
  Morning Glory Breakfast Muffins
      102
  Oatmeal Wheat Bread 110
  Pancakes 105
  Peachy Almond Muffins 105
  Poppy Seed Muffins 104
  Pumpkin Bread 109
  Pumpkin Chip Muffins 104
  Quickie Hamburger Buns 113
  Sweet Muffins 103
  Whole Wheat Cinnamon Rolls
      111
  Whole Wheat Pizza Crust 109
  Zola's Bread 114
  Zucchini Carrot Muffins 106
Brownies
  A.B.C.Brownies 165
  Moist and Chewy Brownies 172
Brown Rice Taco Stack Up 140

Brown Sugar Frosting 186
Brussel Sprouts With Yogurt 120

C

Cabbage and Pineapple Salad 85
Cakes
  Angel Gingerbread 178
  Apple Pudding Cake 179
  Banana Cake 180
  Carrot Cake 181
  Chocolate-Velvet Cake 182
  Fresh Apple Cake With Cinnamon
      Butter 184
  German Chocolate Cake 185
  Oatmeal Cake 186
  Pinto Bean Cake 187
  Pumpkin Nut Cake 188
  Rhubarb Cake 188
Calcutta 56
Cancer: A Learning Process 1
Candy
  Almond Crunch Candy 197
  Cashew Brittle 198
  Creme Caramels 198
  Fruit-Jelly Candies 199
  Maple-Glazed Nuts 199
  Molasses Candy 200
  Penuche 200
  Quick Fudge 201
  Spanish Sweets 201
Caramel Icing 178
Caramel Sour Cream Cookies 168
Carrot-Rice Bake 140
Carrot Cake 181
Cashew Brittle 198
Cashew Honey Butter 67
Celery Pinwheels 57
Cereals
  Apple-Cinnamon Granola 66
  Cranberry-Almond Cereal Mix 69
  Granola 70
  Toasted Granola Surprise 74
Cheese and Broccoli Soup 78

Cherry/Apple Drink 60
Chicken Broccoli Casserole 137
Chicken Noodle Casserole 133
Chili Seasoning Mix 68
Chili Tamale Pie 142
Chilled Fruit Soup 79
Chinese Chews 168
Chinese Sauce 68
Chinese Style Vegetable Medley
      120
Chi Tan Chuan (Chinese Egg Rolls)
      56
Chocolate-Velvet Cake 182
Chocolate Pudding Desert 195
Chuckwagon Beef and Pasta Skillet
      134
Citrus Refresher 60
Cocoa Frosting 183
Coconut-Pecan Frosting 185
Cookies
  Applesauce-Spice Cookies 166
  Basic Sugar Cookies 167
  Caramel Sour Cream Cookies 168
  Chinese Chews 168
  Date Honeys 169
  Easy Does It Cookie Bars 172
  Honey Hermits 170
  Luscious Apricot Squares 171
  Myndy's Chocolate Chip Cook-
      ies 173
  Oatmeal Raisin Cookies 174
  Peanut Butter Crisscrosses 175
  Raw Apple Cookies 176
  Soft Molasses Cookies 177
Cookie Sheet Cake 169
Copper Pennies 121
Cranberry-Almond Cereal Mix 69
Cranberry Blizzard 86
Creamed Peas and Potatoes 121
Creamy Garlic Dressing 158
Creamy Italian Dressing 158
Creamy Tomato Soup 80
Creme Caramels 198

For Health's Sake

Curried Green Beans and Potatoes 122

D

Date Honeys 169
Desert
  Boston Cream Pie 194
  Chocolate Pudding Desert 195
  Flan - French Style 195
  Raisin Apple Betty 196
  Simple Country Cheese Cake 196
  Swiss Strawberry Rice 197
Devilish Eggs 57
Dilly Carrots 123
Dilly Cheddar Muffins 98
Dip
  Guacamole 58
  Nicole's Favorite Herb and Garlic
    Cheese 58
  Seven Layer Bean Dip 55
  Vegetable Dip 60

E

Easy Chili 80
Easy Does It Cookie Bars 172
Egg Substitutes
  Flax Seed Eggs 70
  Unflavored Gelatin Eggs 74

F

Fettuccini and Spinach 143
Fill'er Up Soup 82
Flan - French Style 195
Flax Seed Eggs 70
French-Honey Dressing 159
French Bread 112
French Onion Soup 81
French Tomato Salad 87
Fresh and Fruity 25
Fresh Apple Cake With Cinnamon
    Butter 184
Fresh Strawberry Pie 189

Frosting
  Brown Sugar Frosting 186
  Caramel Icing 178
  Cocoa Frosting 183
  Coconut-Pecan Frosting 185
  Lemon Frosting 183
  Magic Chocolate Frosting 187
  Nutmeg Sauce 179
  Pink Mountain Frosting 183
  Smooth'n Creamy Frosting 181
  Vanilla Cream Filling 182
  White Mountain Frosting 183
Fruit-Jelly Candies 199
Fruit Dishes
  Apple Gratin 117
  Orange Appetizer 117
  Pineapple Boats 118
  Yogurt Fruit Cup 118
Fruit Salad with Orange Poppy Seed
    Dressing 88
Fruit Slushy Mix 69
Fruit Smoothie 61

G

Garden Stir Fry 124
Garlicky Smashed Potatoes and
    Carrots 124
German Chocolate Cake 185
German Chocolate Pie 190
Getting off the Fat-Go-Round 43
Golden Corn Muffins 99
Golden Raisin Buns 100
Good Luck Punch 61
Good Morning Muffins 99
Granny's Whole Wheat Bread 108
Granola 70
Great Web Sites to Check Out 202
Green Beans With Garlic 123
Green Goddess Dressing 159
Guacamole 58

H

Hawaiian Chicken 144

For Health's Sake

Healing the Body and Soul 11
Herbed Oatmeal Pan Bread 107
Herbes de Provence 71
Homestyle Macaroni and Cheese 147
Honey Graham Crackers 101
Honey Hermits 170
Honey Mustard Dressing 160
Honey Pumpkin Pie 191
Hoopla Chicken Lasagna 135
Hot Apple Punch 62
Hot German Potato 87
Humble Pie 145

I

Icebox Butterhorns 108
Index 205
Island Sunset 62
Italian Corn Chowder 81
Italian Dressing 160

L

Lemon Frosting 183
Lemon Fruit Salad Dressing 161
Light and Fruity Salad 89
Light Vegetable Soup With Tortel-lini 82
Luscious Apricot Squares 171

M

Macaroni and Cheese with a Twist 136
Magic Chocolate Frosting 187
Main Dishes
    Amazing Crustless Quiche 138
    Baked Lentils 139
    Brown Rice Taco Stack Up 140
    Carrot-Rice Bake 140
    Chicken Broccoli Casserole 137
    Chicken Noodle Casserole 133
    Chili Tamale Pie 142
    Chuckwagon Beef and Pasta Skil-let 134
    Fettuccini and Spinach 143
    Hawaiian Chicken 144
    Homestyle Macaroni and Cheese 147
    Hoopla Chicken Lasagna 135
    Humble Pie 145
    Macaroni and Cheese with a Twist 136
    Mexican Meatloaf 141
    Mike's Spaghetti Sauce 146
    Mushrooms and Chicken Alfredo 137
    Pepperoni Potato Swirl 149
    Pepper Steak 144
    Sassy Celery Casserole 150
    Seven Layer Dinner 143
    Spanish Rice 141
    Sweet And Sour Pork 148
    Tuna and Rice 151
    Tuna Dressing 151
    Tuna Pasta Salad 138
    Wheat Chili 152
    Zucchini and Pasta 142
Maple-Glazed Nuts 199
Marinated Vegetables 125
Mexican Meatloaf 141
Mike's Spaghetti Sauce 146
Minted Peas 125
Mixes
    Chili Seasoning Mix 68
    Chinese Sauce 68
    Fruit Slushy Mix 69
    Herbes de Provence 71
    Season Salt 71
    Seven Grain Mix 72
    Super Salad Seasoning Mix 72
    Sweetened Condensed Milk 73
    Taco Seasoning Mix 73
Moist and Chewy Brownies 172
Molasses Candy 200
Mooove Over Dairy 39
Morning Glory Breakfast Muffins 102

Mouthwatering Fruit Salad 89
Mushrooms and Chicken Alfredo 137
Myndy's Chocolate Chip Cookies 173
My Good Book List 202

N

Nectarine and Peach Pie 192
New Potatoes with Chopped Mushrooms 126
Nicole's Favorite Herb and Garlic Cheese 58
Norwegian Fruit Salad 90
No Fail Pie Crust 193
Nutmeg Sauce 179

O

Oatmeal Cake 186
Oatmeal Raisin Cookies 174
Oatmeal Wheat Bread 110
Old Fashioned Lemonade 63
Onion-Roasted Potatoes 126
Orange-Apricot Spritzer 63
Orange Appetizer 117
Orange Candied Sweet Potatoes 127
Orange Cream Fruit Salad 90
Oriental Chicken and Vegetable Soup 77

P

Pancakes 105
Parmesan Cauliflower 127
Peachy Almond Muffins 105
Peanut Butter Crisscrosses 175
Penuche 200
Pepperoni Potato Swirl 149
Pepper Steak 144
Pies
  Apple Macaroon 193
  Fresh Strawberry Pie 189

German Chocolate Pie 190
Honey Pumpkin Pie 191
Nectarine and Peach Pie 192
No Fail Pie Crust 193
Pineapple Boats 118
Pink Mountain Frosting 183
Pinto Bean Cake 187
Pizza Sauce 156
Plum Refresher 64
Poppy Seed Muffins 104
Potato-Cheese Soup 84
Potato Chowder 83
Pumpkin Bread 109
Pumpkin Chip Muffins 104
Pumpkin Nut Cake 188

Q

Quickie Hamburger Buns 113
Quickie Salsa 157
Quick Fudge 201

R

Raisin Apple Betty 196
Ranch-Style Buttermilk Salad Dressing 161
Ranch Hand Beans 128
Raw Apple Cookies 176
Raw Cauliflower Salad 91
Refried Beans 129
Rhubarb Cake 188
Rhubarb Slush 64

S

Salads
  Almond Citrus Salad 85
  Ambrosia Platter 86
  Apple Salad 84
  Berry Cream Muffins 98
  Cabbage and Pineapple Salad 85
  Cranberry Blizzard 86
  Dilly Cheddar Muffins 98
  French Tomato Salad 87

For Health's Sake

Fruit Salad with Orange Poppy
   Seed Dressing 88
Golden Corn Muffins 99
Good Morning Muffins 99
Hot German Potato 87
Light and Fruity Salad 89
Mouthwatering Fruit Salad 89
Norwegian Fruit Salad 90
Orange Cream Fruit Salad 90
Raw Cauliflower Salad 91
Salmon Salad Sandwich 91
Tahitian Salad 93
Three Bean Salad 92
Tico Taco Salad 93
Vitamin-Carrot Salad 94
Zucchini Toss 94
Salad Dressing
   Creamy Garlic Dressing 158
   Creamy Italian Dressing 158
   French-Honey Dressing 159
   Green Goddess Dressing 159
   Honey Mustard Dressing 160
   Italian Dressing 160
   Lemon Fruit Salad Dressing 161
   Ranch-Style Buttermilk Salad
      Dressing 161
Salmon Log 59
Salmon Salad Sandwich 91
Sassy Celery Casserole 150
Sauces
   Alfredo Sauce 155
   Barbecue Sauce 156
   Basic White Sauce 155
   Pizza Sauce 156
   Quickie Salsa 157
   Shanni's Hot Fudge Sauce 157
Seasonings by Herb 35
Season Salt 71
Seven Grain Mix 72
Seven Layer Bean Dip 55
Seven Layer Dinner 143
Shanni's Hot Fudge Sauce 157
Simple Country Cheese Cake 196

Smooth'n Creamy Frosting 181
Soft Molasses Cookies 177
Soups
   Ardy's Clam Chowder 77
   Cheese and Broccoli Soup 78
   Chilled Fruit Soup 79
   Creamy Tomato Soup 80
   Cream of Mushroom Soup 79
   Easy Chili 80
   Fill'er Up Soup 82
   French Onion Soup 81
   Italian Corn Chowder 81
   Light Vegetable Soup With Tortel-
      lini 82
   Oriental Chicken and Vegetable
      Soup 77
   Potato-Cheese Soup 84
   Potato Chowder 83
South Seas Corn 129
Spanish Rice 141
Spanish Sweets 201
Stuffed Cucumbers 59
Substitutions, A Guide to 49
Super Salad Seasoning Mix 72
Sweetened Condensed Milk 73
Sweet And Sour Pork 148
Sweet Muffins 103
Swiss Strawberry Rice 197

T

Taco Seasoning Mix 73
Tahitian Salad 93
The Truth about Sweeteners 47
Three Bean Salad 92
Tico Taco Salad 93
Toasted Granola Surprise 74
Toasty Cauliflower and Broccoli
   122
Tropical Fruit Mold 92
Tropical Slush 65
Tuna and Rice 151
Tuna Dressing 151
Tuna Pasta Salad 138

U

Unflavored Gelatin Eggs 74

V

V-7 Juice 65
Vanilla Cream Filling 182
Vegetable Dip 60
Vegetable Dishes
  Baby Carrots with Curry Sauce
      119
  Bean Sprout Casserole 119
  Brussel Sprouts With Yogurt 120
  Chinese Style Vegetable Medley
      120
  Copper Pennies 121
  Creamed Peas and Potatoes 121
  Curried Green Beans and Potatoes
      122
  Dilly Carrots 123
  Garden Stir Fry 124
  Garlicky Smashed Potatoes and
      Carrots 124
  Green Beans With Garlic 123
  Marinated Vegetables 125
  Minted Peas 125
  New Potatoes with Chopped
      Mushrooms 126
  Onion-Roasted Potatoes 126
  Orange Candied Sweet Potatoes
      127
  Parmesan Cauliflower 127
  Ranch Hand Beans 128
  Refried Beans 129
  South Seas Corn 129
  Toasty Cauliflower and Broccoli
      122
Veggie Power 29
Very Berry Cooler 66
Vitamin-Carrot Salad 94

W

Wheat and Other Grains of Knowl-

edge 23
Wheat Chili 152
White Mountain Frosting 183
Whole Wheat Cinnamon Rolls 111
Whole Wheat Pizza Crust 109

Y

Yogurt Fruit Cup 118

Z

Zola's Bread 114
Zucchini and Pasta 142
Zucchini Carrot Muffins 106
Zucchini Toss 94

ABOUT THE AUTHOR

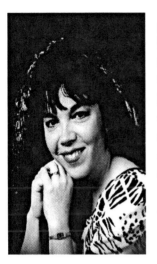

When asked where she is from, MyLinda, generally answers, "What year?" MyLinda Butterworth claims she is no army brat but an education brat. Moving from university to university while her father worked for his higher education. MyLinda is the eldest of eight children, which can explain why she needed all those homemaking skills of cooking, sewing and crafting she learned as a youth. A graduate of Brigham Young University with a degree in Theatre Education, she was prepared to spark the imagination of Junior High and High School students, but opted to help her husband Mike achieve his university education. During that time MyLinda became an award winning costume designer and spent a great deal of time acting, directing and costume designing for a variety of professional and community theatres from Tennessee, Idaho, Arizona and Florida. The majority of her time now is spent raising their children, Nicole and Sean, in the heart of Florida.

In her *spare* time she teaches quilting, thrifty sewing and crafts in the women's organization at her church. She figures since she does't have time to do theatre like she used to, that writing is a new form of creativty. Although the time she generally is allowed to write is between 11pm and 3am, since her children want *all* of mommy's time.

MyLinda claims to be a student of nutrition, one of her passions. She collects, reads and absorbs everything she can find on the subject of nutrtion and cancer. Her husband and children are willing guniea pigs for her tasty creations. And her high energy atests to the fact that what she is doing works.

This is MyLinda's third book. Her first book *For Health's Sake* was written in 1981 on an old typewriter. She produced 500 copies of the book and they were sold by word of mouth (she sold out in 6 months and retired the book). Her second book came out in 1998, *Just 24 Days Till Christmas, Act 1: Old and New* a compilation of stories, activities/crafts and recipes for each of the 24 days leading to Christmas. She has several other books on the horizon, so just keep watching.

Printed in the United States
133270LV00007B/27/A

9 781890 905040